*THE FAMILY IN A
DEMOCRATIC SOCIETY*

THE FAMILY IN A DEMOCRATIC SOCIETY

*Anniversary Papers
of the Community Service Society
of New York*

COLUMBIA UNIVERSITY PRESS · *New York*

1949

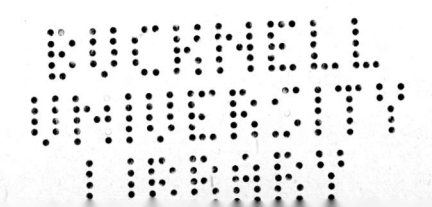

HQ728
.C6

COPYRIGHT 1949, COLUMBIA UNIVERSITY PRESS, NEW YORK

PUBLISHED IN GREAT BRITAIN, CANADA, AND INDIA BY GEOFFREY CUMBERLEGE
OXFORD UNIVERSITY PRESS, LONDON, TORONTO, AND BOMBAY

MANUFACTURED IN THE UNITED STATES OF AMERICA

Foreword

IN OBSERVING its one hundredth anniversary in the spring of 1948, the Community Service Society of New York desired not so much to review the past as to look ahead. Accordingly, the Society offered a program of scientific symposia. These were designed to increase understanding of the present problems of social welfare and contribute to a more effective approach to these problems, by drawing upon knowledge and experience now available in the medical and social sciences and in the practice of social and health work.

The Society had two reasons for welcoming the suggestion that these papers be made more widely available, and in lasting form, through book publication. First, one purpose of our program itself was to bring to a broad public a clearer concept of the place of social welfare in tomorrow's world and thus to strengthen the forces which give impetus to forward-looking social and health programs. Second, many who attended the sessions, and many others who could not come, desired copies of the papers for study.

"The Family in Tomorrow's World" was the theme of this observance since in our belief the family, as the most intimate and influential of all social groups, is the heart of our democratic social order. Part I of this volume includes most of the papers presented at the first symposium, on "Human Relations in Science and Practice." Part II contains the contributions to the second symposium, on "Health and Family Life," in entirety. In another volume, entitled *Social Work as Human Relations*, are published the papers of the third symposium, on "Professional Social Work: Its Substance and World Significance." This marked particularly the fiftieth anniversary of the New York School of Social Work. With them in that volume are the papers presented at the one hundredth anniversary dinner meeting, on "Human Relations in Tomorrow's World," and the balance of the first symposium papers. The sessions were designed for the free interplay of thought and knowledge, and therefore the papers present the views of their individual authors rather than representing necessarily those of the Society or the School.

No introduction to these papers can conclude without expression of gratitude to the authors and to the members of the boards of trustees, of the committees, and of the staffs of the Society and of the School who by their assistance participated in making this historic anniversary observance a significant contribution to the field of social welfare generally. I feel particularly that our whole community is indebted to Walter S. Gifford, chairman of the board, and Bayard F. Pope, president, for the devotion and wisdom of their leadership.

GUY EMERSON, *Chairman*
Committee on the 100th Anniversary,
Community Service Society of New York

New York, New York
March 1, 1949

Contents

Foreword   v
    Guy Emerson

    PART I: THE HUMAN SCIENCES AND THE FAMILY

Variations in the Human Family   3
    Clyde Kluckhohn
Economic Factors in Family Life   12
    Eveline M. Burns
Personal Interaction and Growth in Family Life   29
    Thomas M. French, M.D.
Do We Have a Science of Child Rearing?   41
    John Dollard
Child Rearing in the Class Structure of American Society   56
    W. Allison Davis
Adolescence in Our Society   70
    Harold E. Jones
The Adaptive Problems of the Adolescent Personality   85
    Nathan W. Ackerman, M.D.
Adolescence—Its Implications for Family and Community   121
    Viola W. Bernard, M.D.
Roots of Hostility and Prejudice   141
    Ernst Kris

    PART II: HEALTH AND THE FAMILY

Child Health in Relation to the Family   159
    Martha Eliot, M.D., and Neota Larson

Pioneering in London: the Peckham Experiment INNES H. PEARSE, M.D.	170
Maintenance of Health: Exploring in New York BAILEY B. BURRITT	183
Health and Family Life: Health Maintenance THOMAS D. DUBLIN, M.D., DR.P.H.	194
Constructive Medicine and Positive Health HENRY E. MELENEY, M.D.	198
The Next Generation—Its Nutrition and Health BERTHA S. BURKE	204
Nutrition in the Home and in the Community CHARLES GLEN KING	221
Food for the Family of Nations F. VERZÁR	229
Nursing for Health in Tomorrow's Family RUTH W. HUBBARD	242
Achieving Family Health through Modern Education ERNEST OSBORNE	252
Professional Interplay for Family Health HUGH R. LEAVELL, M.D., DR.P.H.	263
A Public Health Program as a Major Community Service C.-E. A. WINSLOW, DR.P.H.	273
Index of Articles and Contributing Authors	285

Part I: The Human Sciences and the Family

Variations in the Human Family

CLYDE KLUCKHOHN

VARIATIONS IN THE HUMAN FAMILY are interesting and are important both from scientific and from practical standpoints. However, anthropology has tended to overemphasize the differences at the expense of the similarities. Fascinated with the exotic and obsessed with the new principle of cultural relativity, anthropologists have tried to show that the gamut of variability was limitless. Earlier systematic studies seemed to indicate that this was indeed the case. There was the discovery of the extended family system, of the fact that, even in Europe, ultimogeniture existed along with primogeniture; of "visit marriage" in which the man retains residence in his own group. There were those few societies in which two or more men might be married to one woman. But claims for a socially accepted complete promiscuity or for "group marriage" have not stood up under closer scrutiny. And matriarchy, in the strict sense of the term, has turned out to be a myth. What is true is that in some societies the formal and informal power of the mother—both within the family and in political and economic affairs affecting the group as a whole— is greater in some societies than in others. Similarly, the claim that there were groups in which the father had no social relationship to his children is now seen as an extravagant overstatement of a considerable range of variation in the extent of that relationship.

The first generalization to be made, then, is that all variations in the form and functioning of the human family could, until recently, be seen as variations on a basic theme. No aspect of the universal culture pattern has been more clearly delimited than that of the family. The family was always and everywhere an agency for the protection and training of the child and for the care of the aged and the infirm. The manner and extent of this training and care varied considerably, but the basic function was constant. In every society the family was the fundamental institution for the transmission of those patterned ways of living which anthropologists call culture.

The past tense has been used advisedly in the preceding sentences; for the traditional philosophy of the family has been threatened in recent decades. Both in Europe and in the United States the function of protection for the aged, the infirm, and the distressed is being taken over more and more by the State. Greatly increased geographical mobility, changed patterns in regard to employment of married women, and other economic developments make it impossible to regard this long-established functional continuity as still a constant. Under modern urban conditions both men and women can enjoy opportunities (which previously were easily accessible only in family life) without surrendering their independence or assuming family responsibilities.

Every culture legalizes an enduring union between two or more persons of the two sexes explicitly for purposes of parenthood. This nuclear or biological family is never completely submerged in any extended family system. The social approval of sexual union does not in any society constitute in and of itself a marriage or a family. The legitimization of sexuality between husbands and wives, like that prohibition of sexual relations between all other members of the biological family which is an almost constant feature of the human family, is everywhere conceived, not as an end in itself, but as a means to the physical nurture and cultural training of children.

There is nothing mysterious or supernatural about these pan-human regularities in cultural patterns for the family. They bear an understandable relationship to certain inescapable facts in the human situation. Children inevitably go through a period of helplessness. Sickness and old age render adults dependent again. These are biological "givens," which all cultures must face. In the same way it is a biological fact that men are ordinarily stronger physically than women and that women are for longer or shorter periods incapacitated by events of their reproductive cycle. Sexual competition within the immediate family could hardly fail to lead to suffering and to disruption of the family. Hence the restriction of sexuality to husbands and wives may be regarded as one of those aspects of the universal culture pattern that is based upon countless millennia of trial-and-error learning. Exceptions are limited to a few ruling groups and, possibly, to the society of old Iran.

With some qualifications, then, for the contemporary situation in Europe and America, it can be said that there are certain constancies in the functions of the human family. There are also certain regularities in form. The ideal in all human groups has been long-term marriage—though not necessarily between only two partners. The elementary family has ever been conceived as based upon the primary relations of children and parents, with parents related to each other, in the last analysis, through their children. Finally, there are psychological universals. The Freudian description of the Oedipus situation and of sibling rivalry is basically right, even though there are formal variations of this psychological theme; that is, the older person of opposite sex to whom a male child is drawn may be the sister or an aunt, and the older person of the same sex toward whom there exist ambivalent feelings may be an uncle rather than the father. But psychoanalysis has correctly pointed to some inevitable features of the psychodynamics. These words from an Indonesian informant of Cora DuBois suggest one kind of basis for the universality:

Wives are like our mothers. When we were small our mothers fed us. When we are grown, our wives cook for us. If there is something good, they keep it in the pot until we come home. When we were small, we slept with our mothers. When we are grown, we sleep with our wives. Sometimes when we are grown, we wake in the night and call our wives "mother."

It is no accident that in many cultures the term for "sweetheart" is identical with, or similar to, the word for "mother" or "sister."

Within this basic psychological-formal-functional pattern, variations are of three general types. The first may be termed cross-cultural and refers to those differences in blueprints for family living that are standardized as part of the historic tradition of a people. These cross-cultural variations relate in part to the form of the family, in part to its functions.

There are the well-known marriage forms of monogamy, polygyny, and polyandry. These themselves have many variants. While every culture tends to define marriage as ideally permanent, there are many societies, such as our own, in which the behavioral pattern must be realistically described as "serial monogamy." Polygyny ranges from a standard of two or, at most, three wives to the Mohammedan limit of four or the hundreds held by certain African and Asiatic potentates. It is interesting, however, that in these cases only a few women are ordinarily considered wives in the full sense. In some African tribes, for instance, there are only three legal wives—"the head," "the arm," and "the leg" —and the children of concubines are formally ascribed to one of these three. The plural marriage may be to sisters or to nonrelated women or to a woman and her daughter by a previous marriage. In polyandry, also, the marriage of the woman may be to brothers or to nonbrothers. Monogamy, on the whole, appears mainly in the simpler societies and in those where the normal sex ratio is not disturbed. Hobhouse, Wheeler, and Ginsberg found monogamy in only sixty-six societies as against polygyny in 378 and polyandry in thirty-one.

In addition to the marriage pattern, the form of the family is structured by the size of the group included in various social and economic arrangements. The biological family may customarily live alone with the occasional addition of a widowed grandmother or grandfather or collateral relative. Or, the family may be extended to include various relatives on the father's or mother's side of the family or both. Typically, a matrilineal extended family is made up of a grandmother, her husband, her married daughters, their husbands, and their children. In many societies considered matrilineal, however, this typical picture is seldom actualized in all its details. One married daughter lives with her husband's people, or she and her husband and children live as an isolated family unit. One or more sons bring their wives and children to reside with the matrilineal group. In almost every case, membership in what W. Lloyd Warner has called the "family of orientation" continues to some extent when the adult joins in founding a new "family of procreation." Matrilineal, patrilineal, and bilateral families represent ideal types rather than clear-cut forms that apply without qualification to every family in a community.

The forms of family organization prescribed by cultural patterns have consequences that are in the strict sense social rather than cultural. A cultural pattern that provides for sisters and their husbands and children living together in one place determines the nature of interpersonal relations in ways other than dictating economic coöperation, stating that children of sisters shall call each other by sibling terms, behave toward each other as do biological brothers and sisters, etc. The sheer size of the face-to-face group of relatives makes for variation in family life. If the child grows up with a maximum of, say, ten other individuals whom he addresses as "brother" and "sister," the number of personal adjustments he must make is very different from the number that would be necessary in an extended family, where he might have fifty or sixty "brothers" and "sisters." Similarly, any family system involving plural marriages is distinctive, not only because the culture accepts multiple spouses, but also because the interaction rate in a dyadic relationship is different from that in a triadic, tetradic, or still higher set. The addition of each person increases the number of persons in simple arithmetical progression, but the number of personal relations increases in the order of triangular numbers. Of course, this quantitative dimension is enormously complicated by the emotional quality of each given relationship.

It is convenient and in accord with usual practice to restrict the term "family" to that group of relatives who have habitual face-to-face dealings. Thus only the biological families of orientation and procreation and the extended family are included, and such wider units as the clan, phratry, and moiety are excluded. But it should be noted that this conception is an artifact of the Western cultural tradition. The vocabularies of certain nonliterate languages do not include a term that corresponds to our biological family, and some fail even to distinguish the extended family from the whole group of individuals, whether personally known or not, whom one addresses by kinship terms. The distinction between actual mother and mother's sister or classificatory mother can always be and is expressed—when context makes it necessary—by such circumlocutions as "mother from whose body I came" and the like. Yet the concept of a particular group of individuals to whom one's actual biological relations are closest is often not explicit. The secondary parenthood and siblingship implied by a classificatory kinship terminology merges at every point with the relationships we call the "immediate family."

Two family systems can, of course, have approximately the same form but allot the functions within the family organization very differently. The families of the Navaho, Zuñi, and Hopi Indians are all extended, matrilineal, matrilocal. However, the cultural image of the ideal family is not identical in these three cases. The official head of the Navaho family is the father, though emotional and informal authority may actually rest largely with the mother. With the Hopi, authority is, in theory, divided between the mother and her brothers. In practice, the father has a good deal. The Zuñi system falls somewhere between the Navaho and the Hopi. In respects other than that of authority there is also a great and subtle range of variation, both formalized and unformalized. The obligations and expectations of each family member, the tolerated deviations, the stereotypes of ideal role fulfillment—all of these bear a relationship to the formal structure but cannot be predicted solely on the basis of knowledge of the forms.

The second major type of variation may be called the intracultural. In spite of the existence of ideal patterns defining family life for a total society there tend to grow up behavioral patterns that differentiate local or regional groups, economic groups, religious groups, and class groups. In our own society, for example, the existence of a generalized pattern for family organization and behavior is attested by uniformities in the picture

Variations in the Human Family

portrayed in national advertisements, radio programs, and moving pictures. Yet the development of well-established, class-typed family patterns has been shown by Warner, John Dollard, Allison Davis, and others. Among the Navaho polygyny is an accepted pattern of the aboriginal culture. But the actual incidence of polygyny varies widely as between regions where the primary economic base is agricultural, pastoral, or a mixture of these two.

The third principal type of variation may be called idiosyncratic. In no society, however homogeneous, nor in any given segment of that society, is any one family precisely identical with any other. No two individuals play the culturally defined role of mother in precisely the same way. In one family the mother happens, for reasons not culturally controlled, to be much older than the father. To another family the father brings the experience of a previous unhappy marriage. In societies where children are ordinarily born every two or three years, one parent is sterile for a period. Or, if some of the children in a sequence die at an early age, the constellation of that family is unmistakably altered. It is because of a combination of determinants of this order that no particular family ever passes on *"the* culture." Each family transmits its private variant of the culture. And herein lies a fertile source of culture change.

The cause of all these variations in human family life cannot be subsumed in any simple formula. There is some degree of correlation between economic patterns and family organization. Where population density is one to the square mile or less and where livelihood depends on intimate knowledge of the country, the normal form of the family is the simple patrilineal family, with families joined together in bands or hordes. But the correlation is by no means one to one. All kinds of cultural pattern have a way of persisting long after the institutions or circumstances which gave them adaptive value have disappeared. Family patterns may be radically altered as the consequence of widespread acceptance of a new religious cult. This acceptance, in turn, may be determined by a temporary set of economic conditions or other situational factors. Many cultural forms are the product of historical accidents. A variation in family life may, for instance, arise originally as an idiosyncratic variation. A father of a special constitutional type marries a woman who is psychopathic. They manage to work out a form of mutual adjustment for themselves and their children. Most often this particular form would disappear with the end of this particular biological family. But, if the father in question happens to succeed to the chieftainship through the accidental death of his older brother, or if a son of the family founds a new religion, an accidental variant might become the "sacred institution" of a whole people, to be blindly defended and carefully perpetuated.

The practical lessons to be drawn from the foregoing by the applied social scientist (the social worker, for example) would seem to be the following: First, the stuff of human nature is, after all, basically the same because of similarities in human biology and in the conditions of human life. The tailoring is different, and this is significant in making judgments as to how human needs can most effectively be satisfied, as to what incentives will work with one group and not another, as to the meaning of a specific human act. However, the applied social scientist must not be taken in by cultural stereotypes any more than by the simplest, common-sense view of human nature, which is ordinarily a projection of values and beliefs that are local in time and in space. There are patterned variations, whether regional or class or economic, within most cultures. Moreover, there are idiosyncratic variations that sometimes bear only the most general resemblance to the cultural blueprint. In other words, knowledge of a culture or of some segment of that culture can be very useful for general orientation, but one can never expect to drop a perpendicular from the abstracted culture patterns to the behavioral forms existing in a particular family. Finally, the applied social scientist will do well to remember the multifarious causes of variations in human family life. Knowing this, the social worker can steer a difficult but necessary middle course between proper respect for traditional ways of living, as related to the total life design of a group, and absolute acceptance of specific tailorings which usually turn out, after all, to be by-products of adventitious historical events.

Anthropologists have, on the whole, been preoccupied with the more bizarre variations in human family life, such as polyandry. It is now necessary to analyze the subtler differences, to compare, for example, the romantic individualism of American marriage with French marriage which is conceived as a treaty of alliance between two families. What are the formal and functional and psychological differences between family councils of the Chinese and the Japanese type? How do the family patterns of rural Europeans alter after a generation of adaptation to urban life in New York? The case records of social workers are rich in materials for analysis of the answers to such questions as these. Probably social workers are in the best position to make the next advances in our knowledge of variations in the human family.

Economic Factors in Family Life

EVELINE M. BURNS

THE TASK OF THE ECONOMIST who is charged with discussing the economic background against which plans for the future must be worked out is no easy one, for the area is vast. Social development is not discontinuous—what happens in the past influences the present and the future, and if in what follows I shall have occasion to refer to the past, it is because I am searching for clews to the future. Moreover, I shall be very modest in my forecasts. Successful prophecy has, I am afraid, not been one of the outstanding achievements of my profession, though it is true that we have probably been more fortunate in our long- than in our short-run predictions, and 100 years should be a long enough run for anyone.

I propose to concentrate on two major aspects of my subject: (1) the dependence of family well-being upon the continuing flow of a certain minimum of goods and services; and (2) the nature of the economic functions which our society has traditionally assigned to the family. The first of these aspects requires little explanation. We are all too familiar with the adverse and demoralizing effects of inadequate and uncertain incomes upon family life and with the limitations that economic privation places upon the full realization of the rich potentialities of individuals. The second aspect of my subject relates to the fact that in social theory the family as an institution is supposed to discharge a highly important economic function, namely, to provide for the support of those in the productive age groups as well as for the maintenance and training of the new generation and the support of the old. The income to carry out this function is, in turn, assumed to be derived from participation in production on the part of all or some of the adult members of the family group, and the necessity to secure this income is the motivation which society relies on to get its economic work done. This is the theory. One of the questions I shall raise will concern its validity in the light of certain economic developments and trends in social policy.

As we look back on the last 100 years we cannot but be impressed by the vast improvement that has taken place in the economic well-being of the mass of American families. We see this most clearly when we contrast the "untold impoverishment, vagrancy and mendicancy," the utter and apparently hopeless poverty whose existence was the spur to the formation of the Association for Improving the Condition of the Poor in the 1840s, with the condition of those whom we call the "underprivileged" at the present time. It is not merely that, typically, such stark, unrelieved poverty no longer exists, that bare unmitigated poverty is on the way out. Even more significant is the fact that many of our cities and states now define destitution in terms that, had they been operative 100 years ago, would have embraced a substantial part of the working population. Whether we use as our measuring rod the doubling of real earnings between 1840 and 1913 and the subsequent upward trend; or the reduction in average working hours (the time people spend on purely economic activities) from 70.6 in 1850 to 43.0 in 1940; or the general improvement in health and nutritional standards as judged by almost any index we like to use; or the fact that millions of our people are now protected through social security programs against the worst consequences of interruptions to earning power; or the steady increase in the percentage of the population that attend high school or college; or the broadened horizons that are available to families through such gadgets as the automobile, the radio, and the like—only one conclusion is possible: American families, on the whole, are economically much better off than they were 100 years ago. This is not, of course, to say that there are no bad spots. There are many such. The point is that they are "bad spots" rather than generally prevailing conditions, and the "bad" of the 1940s is often better than the "average" or "acceptable" of the 1840s.

The economist would claim that if any one single factor has been responsible for this remarkable improvement in family well-being, it is the enormous increase in America's productivity, reflected in the rise in our national income over these same hundred years. Between 1850 and 1940 our national income (measured in uniform 1940 prices) rose from $4,700,000,000 to $77,600,000,000, or almost seventeenfold. In the same period population increased from 23,200,000 to 131,700,000—somewhat less than a sixfold increase.[1] The average per capita income in 1850 was $207; in 1940 it was almost $580. By 1944, when we were more fully utilizing all our resources, and national income had increased to $122,000,000,000, it had grown to $870 (at 1940 prices). It is the extraordinary increase in output per man hour from 17.3 cents in 1850 to 74.0 cents in 1940 and 79.3 cents in 1944 which has made possible the steady improvement in the living conditions of the vast majority of American families.

At the same time, we must not blind ourselves to the fact that this tremendous increase in economic production has been accompanied by, and indeed in part conditioned upon, certain phenomena which have reacted adversely upon family welfare. It has, in the first place, involved a decline in agriculture and an increase in the importance of industry, commerce, and distribution as the major sources of livelihood. In 1840, 68.6 percent of the labor force was engaged in agricultural pursuits; by 1940 this percentage had fallen to 17.3. This occupational shift has been accompanied by an increasing urbanization of the population. As late as 1880 only 28.6 percent of the population lived in urban areas of 2,500 or more. By 1940, 56.6 percent, or almost double the proportion of our people, were urban dwellers, and the population experts tell us that by 1960 the figure will have risen to almost 60 percent.[2]

---

[1] The figures in this paragraph are derived from J. Frederic Dewhurst and Associates, *America's Needs and Resources* (New York: Twentieth Century Fund, 1947), pp. 23, 32. National income is the value of total net output of goods and services, i.e., the market value of all goods and services produced by private business and government minus all matériel and capital equipment used up in the productive process and all business taxes.

[2] *Ibid.*, pp. 40–41, 620.

Economic Factors in Family Life

At least the first of these trends is a direct concomitant of our success in exploiting modern technology. Both of them have posed new problems. They have gravely interfered with the efficient functioning of the family as the unit responsible for the economic welfare of its members, and notably in regard to the support of the aged. In an agricultural economy and a rural environment the older person, unless completely disabled, was never a wholly nonproductive member of the family group, nor was it an insuperable problem to provide him with shelter and maintenance. Today the situation is far different. Industry, for a variety of reasons, some economically justifiable, some not, discriminates against the older person who is apt to become, from the family point of view, a total economic liability unless his past earnings have permitted adequate savings. The high rents of urban areas, together with the decreasing size of families and changes in consumer tastes, have resulted in smaller housing units which have made it difficult to accommodate the older relative within the household of the active family. Changing economic conditions have thus created in an acute form the problem of the dependent aged. The present generation may justifiably feel somewhat aggrieved at the forces of history which have presented it with this difficult problem precisely at the time when the proportion of aged in the population is increasing so substantially. As against an aged population (age sixty-five and over) of some 10,000,000 at the present time—equal to 12 percent of those between the ages of twenty and sixty-four—we can expect by 1960 an aged population of 14,000,000 and by 1980, 20,000,000, equal to 16 percent and 21 percent, respectively, of the working population in those years.

The shift from agriculture to industry as the typical way of life, coupled with the application of modern technology and large-scale production to agriculture itself, has had yet another adverse effect on the economic welfare of our families. It has meant that an increasing proportion of the population is directly dependent on money income and is less self-sufficient. Any interruption in the continuous flow of this income or in the smooth functioning of the economy as a whole has direct and widespread effects on family well-being. And, unfortunately, our economy has been characterized by very serious dislocations. Over the last hundred years unemployment has become a major threat to the well-being of the vast majority of our families. It is no longer possible to hold that the ability to secure and retain a job is wholly within the control of the individual. As the 1930s have shown, the land is still thought of as providing an ultimate security, and we witnessed the spectacle of millions of the unemployed returning to the farms. But for the vast majority of our people it is no longer possible to tide over periods of interruption to wage income by reliance on home-grown produce. At the same time, this increased dependence on cash income has made our families much more vulnerable to the effects of fluctuations in the general price level.

The trend from rural to urban life has also modified the progress we have achieved, because under urban conditions of living the money costs of securing certain satisfactions are higher than in the rural environment. This is notably the case in recreation. To this extent, therefore, the trend of increased money incomes overestimates the improvement in the economic position of the typical family. Finally, the urban way of life has deprived an increasing proportion of our children of the opportunity for continuous healthy work experience as part of the family group, and our educational system has so far failed to provide an acceptable and effective substitute.

The growth of our national income has, in the third place, been conditioned on a high degree of mobility on the part of the working population, both occupationally and geographically. This economic adaptability of our people is a characteristic of which we often boast, and it is fostered by many of our institutions. Our education system, our training and retraining programs, our employment offices, all encourage mobility, and public opinion is apt to be impatient with families which resist movement from areas of limited, to areas of expanding, job opportunities. And yet this very mobility has adverse and often disastrous effects on family life. The shocking living conditions and the lack of stability and of educational opportunity of the migrant workers of the nation—even in so allegedly progressive a state as New York—

are but the extreme instances of the disrupting effect of geographical mobility upon healthy family life.

More generally, we must recognize too that high mobility further erodes the assumptions on which the older theory of the economic functions of the family was based. For the sense of family cohesion which prompts the spontaneous assumption of responsibility for the support of dependent members is inevitably weakened by the existence of great differences between family members in geographical location or in economic status.

Our highly organized labor market, coupled with the growth of collective bargaining and minimum wage legislation, has resulted in a degree of standardization of wage rates which has greatly intensified the difficulties of those who seek employment but who are disabled or marginally efficient. Furthermore, some share of our increased national income is due to the increase in the number of women who now work in industry rather than in the home. Even by 1940 the proportion of women engaged in paid employment had doubled since 1870, and women now comprise one out of every four instead of one out of every seven gainfully employed. This development too has implications for family well-being.

Our optimism regarding the favorable effect on family welfare of our increasing national productivity must also be modified by another set of considerations. The application of new knowledge has not only resulted in an increase in the number and variety of available products, it has also enabled us to meet old needs in more effective ways, some of which, however, involve the use of costly equipment and highly trained personnel. The concept of adequate and acceptable medical care, for example, is entirely different today from what it was 100 years ago. Unfortunately, the cost of securing it is also completely different. Even if all families shared equally in our higher national income it would still be impossible for the average family to meet from its own income the costs of certain types of medical care.

Finally, we must recognize that the gains from our great increase in national production have not been distributed with reference to need. The statistical measures of the distribution of incomes are still imperfect, but we know that as late as 1941 15 percent of the nation's consumer units (families and single individuals) received cash incomes of less than $500 a year, equal in total to only 2 percent of the total income, while 49 percent received incomes of under $1,500, equal to 19 percent of the total, or less than was received by the 4 percent of the consumer units drawing incomes of $5,000 and over.[3] Income distribution, moreover, is no respecter of size of family. We know, thanks to the studies of Dr. Thomas J. Woofter, Jr.,[4] that almost one third of all American children in 1940 were in families with unit incomes of $150–$299 (an adult counts as a unit; a child as half a unit), and about 70 percent were in families whose unit incomes were below the national median of $474. Dr. Woofter's studies fully document Lord Beveridge's dictum that large families are today a major cause of poverty.

Society has not, of course, remained passive in the face of these challenges to the economic welfare of our families. In fact, the social history of the last 100 years has been the story of the progressive development of conscious control and of social inventions whereby we have aimed to reap the maximum gains from our increasing productivity while protecting ourselves against as many as possible of its adverse consequences. Our approach to the economic problems of families has taken three major forms: First, we have taken measures to increase the money incomes of families. Workers themselves have organized in trade unions to assure that some share of the increasing productivity is reflected in wages. Government has supplemented these efforts by the passage of minimum wage legislation. Other countries have invented and adopted a new social institution, the children's allowance, whereby cash income is paid from the general tax revenues to families, regardless of economic status, in proportion to the number of children in each family.

[3] A recent release indicates that in 1945, 28.6 percent of all families and individuals had total money incomes of less than $1,500; 35.9 percent had between $1,500 and $3,000; 35.6 percent, over $3,000; while 11.9 percent received incomes of $5,000 and over. Bureau of the Census, *Current Population Reports, Consumer Income*. Series P. 60, No. 2. March 2, 1948, p. 11.

[4] Thomas J. Woofter, Jr., "Children and Family Income," *Social Security Bulletin*, January, 1945, pp. 4–9.

Economic Factors in Family Life

Secondly, we have adopted measures to assure the continuity of income, whatever its amount. Here again a new social institution, social insurance, has been brought into being as a method of providing against interruptions of income in a manner which is acceptable to the vast majority of the population because it is free of the invidious associations of the old poor law, of which the needs test has come to be the symbol, and because it has the great advantages of certainty, predictability of amount, and freedom from administrative discretion. The older and parallel institution of public assistance has also been in large measure modernized and reorganized.

The third major line of attack has taken the form of the provision of free or subsidized services and goods. Subsidized consumption has been less used in America than elsewhere. Our subsidized housing program is minuscule and opportunistic. During the 1930s the distribution of surplus commodities formed a substantial part of the income of thousands of American families, but it must be confessed that adoption of the policy was a consequence of the accidental existence of surpluses in the hands of producers: it was not a planned program in which the subsidized items to be distributed were selected by reference to sober consideration of the needs of families. But America's backwardness should not blind us to the fact that subsidized consumption is a powerful technique for increasing the welfare of families, as the example of England today so clearly demonstrates.

In addition to subsidized consumption all modern societies provide certain goods and services free, the costs being met by private philanthropy or from taxation. Education is the outstanding example, but the last hundred years have seen the development, to a lesser degree, of the same policy in regard to health services for certain groups, to family counseling, to recreation. In other countries the provision of free milk and meals to school children, occasionally to be found here, has become a general practice.

As we look ahead to the next hundred years, however, we have many reasons for optimism concerning the economic welfare of American families. First and foremost, the tide of economic development is with us and not against us. Barring the most inexcusable national stupidity there is no reason why we should not be able to maintain and even improve upon the steady increase in productivity which during the past ninety years has averaged 18 percent a decade. The economists and statisticians tell us that the trend of national income is steadily upward, and is likely to increase from the $77,600,000,000 of 1940 to $106,000,000,000 in 1950 and $122,000,000,000 in 1960 (at 1940 prices).[5] This is an increase in income of over 36 percent against a population increase in the same period of 15 percent. Furthermore, we are today the possessors of powerful social tools with which to attack some of the older and more serious obstacles to family well-being, such as the discontinuity of income and the disproportion between family income and size of family. I deliberately refrain, however, from listing our current achievement of full employment among our causes for optimism because of my conviction that the present state of affairs is the result of fortunate accident rather than of any conscious and intelligent social action.

Finally, we have ground for optimism in the fact that we know today much more about the nature of our problem. Economic science, while it has still far to go, has made great strides in the last twenty years, especially in regard to the analysis of the forces making for the greater or lesser utilization of our economic resources, though whether we shall have the courage and fortitude to apply the knowledge is another matter. Moreover, we are armed with a vastly greater body of specific information about the dimensions of the various elements that enter into our problem. If at times we feel overwhelmed by the mass of statistical data and special studies with which the field of social science abounds, and yearn for the simpler days when it was much easier to rate as an expert, we must also remember that this more exact data is a powerful weapon in the fight against ignorance and indifference. We can today meet vague assertions with concrete facts. Even the most complacent of our optimists have been sobered by the statistically revealed fact that in 1935, 25 percent, and in 1941, 15 percent, of the consumer units in the nation existed

---

[5] Dewhurst and Associates, *op. cit.*, p. 23. It should be noted that the frequently quoted figures in Chapter 26 refer to 1944 prices.

on cash incomes of less than $500 a year, especially when, thanks to the development of scientific budget studies, it is possible to give a concrete picture of exactly what such a standard of living means in terms of meals and housing and clothes. Such demonstrations move men to action, where the general statement that "there is still a lot of poverty in the country" leaves them cold. It is less easy to think of those who are dependent on social security income as a class apart when the records show that at the depth of the depression of the 1930s these numbered 28,000,000.[6] Even today there are well over 7,000,000 people dependent for all or part of their livelihood on one or another of our social security programs, not counting the more than 2,500,000 disabled veterans and their families.

More generally, it can be said that those who are concerned about the welfare of families need no longer feel oppressed by the dead weight of abject and uncontrollable poverty. Where it exists today, and extreme poverty still exists in our rich country, it is largely due to our own failure to take full advantage of our available social controls and our new social welfare techniques.

But all this does not mean that from now on we can sit back with folded hands thankful that the problem of poverty has been overcome. On the contrary, there is still much to do, and new challenges to our ingenuity and our courage face us. It will be obvious from what I have just said that we have still to exploit to the full the social techniques at our disposal. In the economic field we have yet to complete the reform of our social security system. At the very least, we should bring it up to the levels that other countries, notably Great Britain and New Zealand, have achieved. It is a shameful fact that we in America cannot yet say that every American has access to some form of basic economic security whether it be through social insurance or public assistance. In the course of the next hundred years, too, we shall have to tackle the problem of the economic position of members of large, or moderately large, families. I am not as yet sure that we could take over the institution of children's allowances in its en-

[6] *Security Work and Relief Policies* (National Resources Planning Board: United States Government Printing Office, Washington, D.C., 1942), p. 445 and Appendix G.

tirety, though this has proved valuable elsewhere. But whether we handle the problem through this method or through an expansion of subsidized consumption, or by free goods and services, or by some as yet uninvented social technique, the problem is one we cannot evade if we care about the economic welfare of families. Here again, it is curious that America, whose interest in child welfare is world renowned, should have been so neglectful of this aspect of family well-being and so unresponsive to the astonishing progress that has been made in other countries in recent years. In my view, it should be one of the major items on our agenda for the next hundred years.

Furthermore, we must more vigorously tackle certain of the less desirable by-products of our progress to which I have already referred. The income problem of the aged can undoubtedly be attacked through techniques already at our disposal, though there are still some issues we have not yet fully resolved, such as the question of the appropriate living standard for such a large nonproductive segment of the population, and the question of whether our social policies should be devised to encourage or discourage people from working after a certain age. But we must also remember that income security is only one element in the welfare of this large group, and the economic developments I have sketched bring, in their turn, other and as yet unsolved problems of housing, personal services, and appropriate occupation during the years beyond sixty-five that science is continually prolonging. Similarly, in the next hundred years we must discover some means of enabling the average family to secure those services, notably medical and psychiatric care, whose cost is prohibitive if concentrated on the individual but bearable if spread among all those exposed to the risk.

The growth of our national income and the degree of success we have already achieved in the abolition of the direst forms of poverty, in turn, present us with new challenges; for in the course of years our concept of poverty has itself changed. We can say that our measure of what constitutes an acceptable minimum standard of living has become more liberal. It is here that we must be alert to see that there is no unjustifiable lag, either in the revision of that standard as the wealth of the country increases, or in its incorporation into public policy. The standard of living for recipients of public or private aid that was acceptable in 1900, when the national income was $345 per capita, will not be appropriate in 1950 when the income per capita will average $730 (at 1940 prices).

We must be on the alert to raise our sights in yet another way. In the measure that we succeed in preventing families from falling below the prevailing acceptable minimum standard of living, we must shift from a concern about the so-called "underprivileged" to a concern about the living conditions of a much wider segment of the population. For even this minimum level of health and decency is nothing to boast about, and immediately above it there exists a large population group whose standard of living still falls short of what is consistent with our high levels of national output. We must be beware of being unduly influenced by the historical fact that welfare activities originally centered in the so-called "destitute" groups if only because of the social undesirability and popular unacceptability of a policy which provides superior services of a kind needed by the population as a whole, primarily to one group, and that a group dependent on socially provided income. The next hundred years must see a new area of operation, calling for new social tools appropriate to the larger numbers involved so that it will no longer be said, for example, that "only the very rich and the very poor can get good medical care."

Yet another major challenge faces us in the years that lie ahead. It is evident from what I have already said that the upward trend of national income will not automatically and inevitably involve a corresponding improvement in the economic well-being of the mass of our families. Indeed, alone, it will not even insure that all families will be buoyed up to the basic minimum living standard. The Twentieth Century Fund's economists tell us that even the much higher levels of income of the 1950s and 1960s will leave a large fraction of American families with income inadequate to buy enough of the necessities of life to maintain themselves at a health and decency level. More specifically, if the consumption of those above this level is not to be modified, we would require 11 percent more goods and services in 1950 and 7 percent more in 1960 than is provided for even at the higher levels of income expected to prevail in those years. The main deficits occur in foods, though housing, medical care, and household operation also bulk large.

Furthermore, we must not forget that if these needs are to be met there must be a considerable expansion of capital facilities and that above the health and decency minimum, even a modest estimate of the needs of consumers for housing, education, public welfare services, and the like, would call for expenditures substantially larger than could be met within the higher national incomes of 1950 or 1960. Thus we still face the essential economic problem of making the best use of limited resources despite our higher levels of productivity. As in the past, those who care about the welfare of the American family will have to insist that if there is a limit to what we can have, first things must come first.

In this context the social policies we have adopted for maximizing family welfare meet very real obstacles and for two reasons. First, they involve competing claims upon the total national production; a demand, for example, that relatively more resources be devoted to increasing the total of domestic consumption. Here we run up against other major claims upon our total resources. Today these other claims on national income are formidable. Some part of our resources must at all times be devoted to increasing our investment in trained personnel and accumulation of capital equipment, for it is on the continuance of this activity that our rising production curve depends. In America, it seems likely that this competing claim will not prove a severe limitation to our ability to raise living standards, though its existence must never be forgotten. In England, however, the situation is far different: a much poorer country, which has done much more than we have to insure the basic minimum to all its citizens, is today forced to choose between building houses and hospitals on the one hand, and re-equipping its all-important export industries on the other—and has courageously chosen the latter.

Much more serious in the years that lie ahead will be the competing claims on our large but limited resources exerted by armament expenditure and the potential of foreign relief and reconstruction. A few years ago many of our economists were worrying about ways and means of insuring a continuing demand for our large potential economic output, and were, *inter alia,* hoping and planning for an expansion of the social services as a method of taking up the slack. They reckoned without the armed forces, whose current estimates of minimum needs would create a demand for a much larger proportion of our total output than was even suggested in the most inflated estimates of possible social expenditures! The estimates I have given of the higher but still inadequate levels of consumption permitted by the national income of the future assumed that only six or seven billion dollars would be devoted to military expenditure. Obviously, the share available for increasing family well-being will be greatly reduced by the 1948 defense budget which more than doubles that sum, let alone what it will be if our military friends who envisage expenditures of twenty to forty billions have their way.

Secondly, within the limits of that segment of total national output devoted to current consumption it seems probable that in the forecastable future the substandard families will be raised to the acceptable minimum only by a continuance of the three types of social policy we have evolved during the last century, namely, direct transfers of income from the richer to the poorer, an expansion of subsidized consumption, and an extension of the social insurance technique. These measures have in common the fact that for a very large proportion of Americans they involve a compulsory curtailment of freely disposable income, meaning thereby that portion of income which a man can spend as he likes after payment of taxes and other demands on him which are almost equally compulsive. (Contributions to community chest drives sometimes fall in this category.) Another of the main items on our agenda for the future, therefore, will be finding ways in which to persuade the average income receiver to continue to support measures which may or may not benefit him directly, but which certainly cut into his freely disposable income.

Part of the opposition to public and private welfare programs, even when they benefit him, lies in the average man's conviction that he knows better than does any public or private agency what kinds of expenditure give him satisfaction. A nation which today spends more than twice as much money for liquor and tobacco as for medical care, about the same for movies as for support of the Church, and almost as much for beauty parlor services as for private social welfare will not easily be convinced of the desirability of sacrificing some of what Mrs. Sidney Webb once referred to as "men's silly pleasures" in return for more adequate medical or psychiatric care, free milk for school children, or better staffed and equipped schools. In this connection it is difficult to feel that the agencies responsible for the welfare of families have in recent years devoted enough attention to narrowing the gap between their own conception of minimum family needs and that which is held in practice by a large majority of the voters and potential givers. The present state of affairs calls, among other things, for a vigorous re-examination by the agencies themselves of their own standards in terms both of their relationship to the values held by the average man and woman, and of their realistic practicability in a world of increasing but still limited economic output.

Some further part of the opposition on the part of the taxpayer or philanthropic giver is also attributable to a suspicion on his part that the funds of agencies, whether public or private, are not always spent in the most economical manner. Here again we who are concerned with family welfare are not wholly blameless. It would be a bold person who would assert that the maximum effectiveness is today secured from the substantial sums devoted to private welfare in our communities. On the contrary, we see overlapping of function, maintenance of vested interests, and a lamentable failure to consider total needs in relation to total resources and to allocate funds in such a way as to give priority to the most urgent needs. Our public agencies, too, although their activities are more exposed to the limelight of public knowledge and criticism, have equally failed to convince the average taxpayer that they keep a proper balance between his interests and those of the public welfare client.

But beyond these more obvious reasons, I suspect a deeper and more subtle reason for the opposition of the taxpayer to further inroads into his freely disposable income for welfare purposes and for the resistance of the private giver to the drive for funds for private welfare. It lies, if I am correct, in a very real uncertainty as to the philosophical basis of the whole welfare policy. And here I return to the theory of the economic functions of the family. Officially, and as a nation, we still retain the traditional theory that the family is responsible for the economic welfare of its members, and that this responsibility is the spur which goads men and women to seek and retain employment. A policy which softens the impact of unemployment, which brings an increasing flow of free or subsidized goods and services to the family, and which tends to relieve it of certain traditional economic responsibilities, notably in regard to children and the aged, necessarily challenges this whole philosophy. Hitherto, nothing has been put in its place—and what must perhaps be even more confusing to the average man or woman, our practical departures from the older theory have been neither logical nor consistent.

Why, for example, do we retain the needs test for some types of social security income and dispense with it for others? None of our rationalizations satisfies the man who sees his neighbor entitled to unemployment compensation for which he has paid no contribution, but finds himself excluded merely because he works for a small firm or a nonprofit agency. What must be the feelings of the man who, firmly believing in the traditional theory, determines to rely solely on his own efforts and sees a possibly irresponsible neighbor not merely supported out of tax funds, but, because of his dependent status, receiving services which he too would like, but cannot afford? Who can make any sense of the different standards of need that prevail in the various public and private social services in any one city? Why do we admit that children are an economic liability for those rich enough to pay income taxes, but disregard this fact in relation to those too poor even to pay such taxes? Is it even intelligent for a society which lays so much stress on the formative influence of childhood years to develop a social security program which treats children so much less favorably than the aged? I suggest that it is not surprising that the average citizen is confused about our purposes and our philosophy.

It is not enough to say that the man who opposes further inroads on his freely disposable income has an outmoded social philosophy or that social workers have fallen down on the job of interpretation. The fundamental difficulty is the lack of a realistic modern philosophy to replace the old. Somehow, during the next hundred years, we must evolve a reformulation of the economic functions of the family which will be based upon the economic and social realities of the twentieth century. It must embrace, too, a theory of economic incentive which, while rejecting the assumption that starvation is the only spur to participation in production or that man works only for economic reasons, will also reject the equally unrealistic assumption that all men are spontaneously coöperative angels—or would be if only they were all psychoanalyzed.

The job is nothing less than a consistent reformulation of the mutual rights and responsibilities of the individual, of the family, and of organized society. As I contemplate the future, I will venture at least one prophecy: the job to be done in both theory and action in connection with the economic welfare of the family is still so great that those of us whose minds and time are given to this task will certainly have no reason to fear the old economic bugbear of technological unemployment.

Personal Interaction and Growth in Family Life

THOMAS M. FRENCH, M.D.

PSYCHIATRISTS ORDINARILY DEAL with the problems of an individual in adapting to his social environment. A psychiatrist's responsibility to his patient compels him to view one-sidedly a problem in group adjustment. But the adjustment of one individual to a group is only a part of a more comprehensive adaptive process, of the process of mutual adjustment of the members of the group to each other.

For the family agency, it is the family rather than the individual that is the unit. A psychiatrist who works with a family agency soon finds himself under pressure to retranslate his knowledge into new terms. He has been accustomed to study problems of social adjustment from the point of view of the interest of his own particular patient but in a family agency he must develop a new orientation. He can no longer center his interest upon the needs of one individual but must study how the needs of the different members of the family group can best be reconciled.

In recent years clinical psychiatry too has been undergoing a reorientation that makes this task somewhat easier. There was a time when psychoanalytic psychiatry was interested primarily in explaining disturbing symptoms, when it sought its explanations first of all in disturbing motives that the patient's ego had rejected and repressed. This was a necessary stage in the development of our knowledge; for the scientific world, as well as society in general, resisted frank recognition and discussion of disturbing sexual and hostile motives, and this was an obstacle that had to be overcome before any scientific understanding of the psychoneuroses and psychoses could be possible at all. But after he had broken through this barrier, Freud turned his attention to the other side of the problem—to a study of the defenses employed by the ego to protect itself from disturbing wishes. It was at this time that psychoanalysis first became really interested in the conscience, and in the sense of guilt and the need for punishment with which the conscience often protests against forbidden wishes.

Guilt is not the only motive that puts pressure upon the ego to repudiate disturbing impulses. The inhibiting motive may be fear, or pride, or fear of offending some loved person. Now that we have become interested successively in each side of a conflict, a still more comprehensive approach becomes possible. We can begin to view the conflict as a whole, as a problem that requires solution. Psychoanalytic psychiatry is now becoming interested in the problem-solving or integrative function of the ego, in questions of how the ego struggles to find a way of reconciling conflicting motives.

The transition from a psychiatry oriented to the needs of an individual to a psychiatric understanding of mutual adjustment within a group is really very similar to the transition that we have just described. Now that psychiatry has attained some proficiency in studying problems of social adaptation from the point of view of the needs of one individual, it can next study two or more members of a group successively and then utilize the understanding thus gained to attack the more comprehensive problem of how the members can adjust to each other.

It is already widely recognized that in order to understand the emotional problems of a child it is usually necessary to understand those of the parents also. Often, in order to help the child, we must treat one or both parents. Thus in child psychiatry we are already beginning to think of the family as a social unit and to look upon the maturation and adjustment of any one individual as part of a process of mutual adjustment within a group.

In marital conflicts the problem is, of course, quite frankly one of mutual adjustment. Only too often the psychiatrist finds himself unable to help much in marital conflicts because either one or both partners can see the problem only in terms of his or her own needs and of his desire to make over the other to suit these needs. When we succeed in contributing to the solution of marital difficulties it is usually because we have been able to help the two partners to a better mutual understanding of each other's needs. We succeed best when each is able to develop the same understanding tolerance for the other that the psychiatrist must acquire toward the disturbing wishes and impulses of his patients.

One of the most important characteristics of all life is change. Human life especially is a long series of readjustments to changing situations. The best way to study individual development is to reconstruct the problem involved in each readjustment; and a disturbance in emotional equilibrium can best be understood by studying it as a failure to solve a problem in readjustment.

In the last fifty years a great mass of information has been accumulated and analyzed, throwing light on most of the typical processes of readjustment that occur in the lives of the great majority of individuals in our culture. Now, by putting together what we know about individual development it is possible also to get some understanding of the typical mutual readjustments that take place in family life.

Since we have to choose a starting point, let us consider first the readjustments that are set in motion by the expected birth of a new individual. We do not always realize that the nine months of pregnancy, especially in the case of the first child, are a period of emotional preparation and readjustment for both prospective parents. This is particularly true for the prospective mother, of course. I suspect that no one has ever faced the prospect of becoming a parent entirely without conflict. A new child threatens so many old adjustments! If there is any lingering longing to be loved oneself as a child, then the expected baby revives latent conflicts from the time when the expectant mother or father once had to accept a newcomer in the parental home. Then too, the newly married couple have perhaps just been getting used to having each other all to themselves and may be expected to resent sharing each other's love with a child.

It is not possible to give up an old gratification unless one can find a new one to take its place. We owe to Freud a beautiful delineation of what is probably the chief source of satisfaction in playing the role of parent, a satisfaction which normally goes far to recompense the parent for renouncing more dependent and self-centered cravings, as his or her new role requires him to do:

If we look at the attitude of fond parents towards their children, we cannot but perceive it as a revival and reproduction of their own, long since abandoned narcissism. . . . Thus they are impelled to ascribe to the child all manner of perfections which sober observation would not confirm, to gloss over and forget all his shortcomings . . . they are inclined to suspend in the child's favor the operation of all those cultural acquirements which their own narcissism has been forced to respect, and to renew in his person the claims for privileges which were long ago given up by themselves. The child shall have things better than his parents; he shall not be subject to the necessities which they have recognized as dominating life. Illness, death, renunciation of enjoyment, restrictions on his own will, are not to touch him; the laws of nature, like those of society, are to be abrogated in his favor; he is really to be the centre and heart of creation, "His Majesty the Baby," as once we fancied ourselves to be. He is to fulfill those dreams and wishes of his parents which they never carried out, to become a great man and a hero in his father's stead, or to marry a prince as a tardy compensation to the mother. . . . Parental love, which is so touching and at bottom so childish, is nothing but parental narcissism born again, and transformed though it be into object-love, it reveals its former character infallibly.[1]

A case which was reported at one of the conferences of the United Charities in Chicago will illustrate, not only the problem involved in this step in readjustment, but also some aspects of the next readjustment that the fond parent will be called upon to make. The client was a young married woman in her middle twenties, who had already had several children and was continually becoming pregnant although her husband was very inadequate and always out of work. She got some advice about contraceptives but was extremely careless about carrying it out and confessed to a compulsive fascination for taking care of little babies which undoubtedly played an important role in motivating her pregnancies. But unfortunately for the children that she

[1] Sigmund Freud, *Collected Papers* (London: Hogarth, 1934), IV, 48–49.

brought into the world in this way, after a few years her passionate tenderness toward them was followed by loss of interest, and neglect, and by a compulsion to get another baby upon whom to bestow her devotion.

We were, of course, interested to inquire how the young woman had developed this rather bizarre exaggeration and distortion of the maternal urge. She was the oldest of three children, and she told us that for five years her own parents had made her the center of the family circle. But then came twin sisters, and our patient felt utterly neglected.

We cannot fail to be impressed by this parallel between the patient's own behavior and her subjective memory of how she was treated by her parents. But one who studies a patient's reactions as attempts at readjustment will not be quite satisfied with this answer. It is evident that the birth of the baby sisters must have been an intensely frustrating experience. In reaction to this frustration we should expect that she would have developed intense resentments toward her rivals and probably strong guilt feelings. This is the reaction that we most frequently encounter in children when the birth of a younger child has played such a traumatic role. But this young woman has developed a passionate delight in taking care of little babies. We believe that the capacity to find such delight in giving love cannot be accounted for merely as a compensatory reaction to hostility and guilt but must have its basis in the child's having received some compensatory form of love at the time that it was so much needed. Our expectation was confirmed in this particular patient's case. When we raised the question, the worker responsible for the case told us that the little girl had not felt completely neglected when the parents turned their affection from her to the baby sisters but had herself turned to her grandfather, who lived in the home and whose favorite she continued to be.

But there is a wide gap between the birth of the baby sisters and the time when the patient developed a compulsion to take care of little babies. What form did the patient's compensation take when she was five years old, at the time when she turned to her grandfather for the affection that she was no longer receiving from her parents? At this point we hazarded a guess. We guessed that there must have been a doll in the story, that she and her grandfather must have played with great intensity at taking care of this doll "baby." At the time of the conference the worker did not know whether this guess was correct, but at the next conference he reported that the little girl had had a baby carriage which she kept until she married and a doll with which she slept until she was grown.

This story illustrates dramatically the role played by a parent's identification with her child to compensate for renunciation of her own craving to be loved as a child. In this case the birth of younger babies demanded this renunciation too soon from an older sister who was herself still only a child.

This patient's behavior also illustrates two other points that we must grasp if we wish to understand what makes this kind of readjustment possible. First we notice that vicarious gratification of her need to be the center of her parents' affection was made possible for this little girl only by her grandfather's continued devotion. In the usual emotional readjustment of an expectant mother to her pregnancy and to the child after it is born, she normally receives very much needed emotional support from her husband's love and from his participation in a common pride and delight in their plans for the coming baby. The grandfather's participation in our patient's fantasies about her doll baby is only an exaggerated version of this normal role of the child's father in the emotional readjustment that makes it possible for a young mother to accept vicarious gratification for her own dependent needs by devoting herself to the baby.

This patient's story illustrates also difficulties that may ensue when this kind of adaptation to the needs of the child ceases to be adequate. The young woman's need to be compensated for renunciation of her own babyhood paradise was so great that she was quite unable to readjust to the child's changing needs when it ceased to be a baby. Her compulsion was devotion to little babies. As soon as the child grew older she lost interest in it.

A similar difficulty in adjusting to the changing needs of the child is not infrequently encountered somewhat later in the child's life. Sometimes parents demand that the child fulfill their own frustrated ambitions instead of choosing a career that the child's own interest dictates. A father who has been disappointed in his own ambition to become a physician may insist upon putting his child through medical school, in spite of the fact that the child's own spontaneous interests are artistic rather than technical and that the child himself may wish to be an artist or an architect rather than a physician. Thus if the need for vicarious gratification is too importunate, a parent may find it quite impossible to adapt himself to the changing needs of the child.

A more normal parent will not be so fixed on any one memory of happiness in childhood but will have a rich store of memories to deepen his or her understanding of the child and to make it possible to participate in and enjoy vicariously each phase of the child's development.

If the child develops normally he will be called upon to make a long series of very important readjustments. The infant starts life as "His Majesty the Baby," who is given love and care without anything being expected of him in return. But in the course of the next few years:

1. If he wishes to be loved, as of course we all do, he must learn to please others, to win love, to win the mother's or father's approval by doing what the parents tell him to do, by being a "good" child.

2. He will be expected in gradually increasing degree to take care of his own needs instead of expecting others to take care of them, accepting pride in achievement in place of the desire to be cared for.

3. He must adjust himself to the fact that there are some things that one cannot have at all and others for which one must wait, or wait and strive, accepting for a time the joys of anticipation in place of those of immediate gratification.

The necessity for all these readjustments is likely to be forced upon him with particular suddenness by two events.

1. The birth of another child will face the older child with the necessity of sharing the love and care that he has perhaps felt previously to be his own exclusive right. Indeed, the new baby, since

it is younger, will almost certainly receive more care and attention, and the older child will be compelled to win the love and approval that he desires by adapting his behavior to the parents' demands, or to accept pride in achievement in place of his desire to compete with the baby as a helpless infant.

2. When he goes to school, still more will be expected of him in both these ways. He will have to share the teacher's interest with the whole classroom full of children of his own age; and he will probably not get the teacher's love for nothing but will have to earn her approval by achievement and good behavior. Many of the difficulties that some children have when they first go to school are based upon their rebellion and protest at being expected to make these two kinds of readjustment.

It is, of course, the parents who must exert much of the pressure that forces the child out of the patterns of babyhood into those expected of an older child. This obviously requires emotional adjustment on the part of the parents. Since many of the child's undisciplined impulses interfere with the comfort and convenience of the parents, their own annoyance will sometimes reinforce the demands of custom and of the community at large that the child be made to conform. But it is unfortunate, if a parent fails to distinguish carefully between his own convenience and his task to train the child in habits that will make possible the child's gradual assimilation into the wider community.

A number of other possible motives may cause a parent to overdo the task of imposing discipline upon a child. A father may himself have been too strictly or severely disciplined and may take a kind of revenge upon the child for what he suffered in his own childhood. Or the parent may have had difficulty in self-discipline in relation to some particular kind of forbidden impulses and may react with panic and desperation if the child shows even slight tendencies in the same direction. In such a case the child, reacting to the parent's desperation, will almost certainly become fixated upon a conflict similar to the parent's. Or if the father is a strong and dominant personality and unable to soften his discipline with an understanding interest in encourag-

Interaction and Growth in Family Life 37

ing his son's spontaneity, the son may be helpless to assert himself against his too powerful father and may be seriously inhibited in developing independence and initiative. In other cases the father may need to assert his authority against his relatively helpless child for exactly the opposite reason, as a compensation for his own sense of weakness.

At the other extreme are parents who overreact to their aggressive impulses against their children by inability to discipline them, or who identify too intensely with their children's more dependent needs and therefore require too little of them.

The needs and problems of children vary so widely that it is quite impossible within present limitations to discuss at all exhaustively the attitudes in the parents that are most conducive to the healthy development of their children or the still more basic question as to what influences in the parents' background and experience may make it possible for them to acquire these desirable attitudes. But one point is becoming increasingly widely recognized as a result of the present growing intcrest in the emotional development of the child. This is the need for sensitive and sympathetic understanding of the child's behavior and of what motivates the child's reactions to the discipline that must be imposed upon it. Only under the guidance of such understanding can a parent perform his or her task of child training intelligently. How one can acquire such a capacity for understanding a child, and what kind of satisfactions will reward those who are successful in achieving such understanding are topics of too wide scope to be discussed profitably at this time.

Let us now consider some of the problems of adolescence which can so easily upset the equilibrium of the whole family. The intensification of sexual urges that comes with puberty gives rise to problems that are likely to be very perplexing and disturbing, not only to the maturing child but to the parents as well. These impulses are perplexing and disturbing for two reasons: (1) they are apt to run counter to parental and social prohibitions; and (2) they force upon the child even more acutely the problem of adjusting his or her needs, first, to the equally pressing needs of another and different individual and then to the biological fact that these cravings tend inevitably to bring new problems with them in the form of children.

It has been customary in our culture to treat the problems of adolescence primarily as disciplinary problems, and to center attention upon parental and social prohibitions rather than upon the adolescent's new problems of adjusting to another individual and of taking on responsibility for a family, that the sexual urges usually bring in their train. But it is these latter problems that are most important for the future development of the adolescent. In recent years social agencies have been devoting attention increasingly to the problems of unmarried mothers; and one thing that these studies bring out most clearly is the fact that too energetic condemnation and inhibition of sexual urges leaves the young girl totally unprepared for the responsibilities and the problems of mutual adjustment, in which she will find herself involved when these sexual impulses do finally break through or are permitted to emerge. Mother Nature is so intent upon getting the race reproduced in spite of all obstacles that she permits young girls, in response often to very childish motives, to become involved quite unwittingly in the responsibilities of parenthood. The boys, of course, fare better since Mother Nature permits them, if they wish, to run away from their responsibilities; society has found great difficulty in compelling unwilling fathers to share the burden that they help to create.

Our studies show that the most important single factor in the preparation of the young woman for motherhood is her relationship to her own mother during the difficult years of adolescence. We have already pointed out how parental love has its firmest basis in memories of the love that the expectant parent herself once received as a child. This same security in a mother's love should now protect the adolescent girl from turning too precipitately to seek outside the affection that she does not receive at home. Our studies of unmarried mothers show that the unreflecting, popular concept of these problems gives us a very inadequate picture. It is not always or only uncontrollable sexual urges that drive these girls into ill-considered relationships with men.

Over and over again we discover that the girl in turning to men is seeking, too naïvely, a substitute for parental love, when she feels that her own mother or a maternal older sister has failed her. I recall in particular a young girl who dreamed of riding through the streets in a dirty wagon and soiling her own pure white dress when she learned that her mother was involved in an illicit sexual relationship. Soon afterward the girl herself became illegitimately pregnant.

Inhibition and restraint of too importunate sexual urges are only a temporary and secondary part of the mother's proper role in relation to her daughter. Adolescence is an experimental period when boys and girls learn to know what to expect from each other. It is a time when both boys and girls should be learning to integrate their impulsive attraction for each other with a knowledge of probable consequences. Strong sexual cravings and longings to receive and give love need to be synthesized with discriminating appraisal of the motives and reliability of the men to whom the young woman is attracted, and with frank willingness to undertake the maternal responsibilities in which her sexual urges will probably soon involve her. She must learn to protect herself against letting Mother Nature trick her into becoming unwillingly committed to responsibilities which she is not yet ready to accept. The girl's mother has presumably had some experience in these matters. If her relationship with her daughter is sufficiently confidential, she should be able to help the daughter anticipate some of the consequences of her impulses and thus protect her from having to learn from bitter experience. We often do not appreciate the constructive value of the fantasy activity in which this period is so rich. These fantasies have potential educational value, enabling the young girl or boy to live through in imagination many things that he or she is not yet prepared to live through in real life. A wise mother whose relationship with her daughter is such as to permit her to become acquainted in this way with the daughter's more intimate aspirations can be of great service in helping her to anticipate in imagination and digest emotionally consequences that will later have to be faced in real life.

But the time should come when this task too is completed. We may perhaps best conclude this discussion by looking forward for a moment to the next readjustment that life will demand of the mother. Even the joys of responsible adult life must one day be renounced. The children grow up and must be allowed to live their own lives. Perhaps nowhere is the need for wise prophylaxis greater than in anticipation of this time, when life will become very empty unless a mother has taken care to cultivate other interests which can continue to make life rich even after the responsibilities and joys of parenthood have been fulfilled. For the husband and father this readjustment is often easier because he still has his work outside the home. But he too will do well to find other satisfactions to make life worth while when younger men press forward to take over at least part of the roles that he has been accustomed to play.

Do We Have a Science of Child Rearing?

JOHN DOLLARD

A HUNDRED YEARS AGO there was much of wisdom and compassion written concerning children. The names of Locke, Rousseau, Pestalozzi, and Montessori come to mind. But there was no Freud—father or daughter; no Ferenczi, no Abraham, no Binet, no Goddard, no Mead nor Watson; no Kluckhohn nor Piaget; no Gesell nor Anderson; and no Pasteur—to call only a few of the roll of hundreds of shining names. Truly, a hundred years has done much for children. Searching, sweat, and genius have piled up their innovations of fact and imagination to create a new perspective on the child and, indeed, on human personality itself.

It was natural that the physical growth of the child should be studied first, and much has been learned in this field. Scientists grasped first at the measurement devices which were readily available. They turned out to be the calipers, the ruler, the X-ray, and with these instruments those characteristics were measured which could thus be measured. Thousands of papers in various journals and scientific fields attest the vitality of anthropometry.

Binet set out in a new direction. He guessed that children could be sorted into various groups on the basis of their responses to certain realistic problem stimuli, and he devised such sets of problems. This was an attempt, not merely to borrow the measuring instrument from another discipline, but to fabricate a special one of relevance to the problem at hand. His notion of "mental age" was soon transformed into mental age over chronological age, giving rise to the intelligence quotient—a means of ranking children of any age in respect to the mean accomplishment of children of the same age. The intelligence quotient has been immensely serviceable. It and similar indices have provided a means of sorting whole populations into groups with relation to particular tasks, have aided in psychiatric diagnosis, and have encouraged the intelligent social treatment of the little gifted.

Problems in this field have, again, given rise to a great literature, much of it centered on the question of the consistency of the intelligence quotient. There seems little doubt nowadays that there is a great deal of consistency in the mental growth career of an individual. This may be due to somatic pattern, to a fortunate start with advantage maintained, to superior environmental conditions, or to some combination of all of these. In this connection some writers have stressed the importance of a "critical period" for the emergence of certain phenomena. If the opportune moment be lost, the child or animal may lag in development and never accomplish the missing units.

In the field of child research certain standard debates have been formulated which have been productive in getting critical work done. One of these debates relates to how early and in what respects the child can be conditioned, though it must be admitted that such debates generate a considerable fog as well as some clarification. It seems likely that the infant is conditionable in some respects soon after birth and that we do not need to suppose that learning awaits some advanced stage of neural maturation. The responses which can be learned are, however, simple, and only a technician can perceive their importance in relation to the eventual complex structure of human behavior.

The issue of maturation versus practice has also received much scientific attention. So far as the available data go, it seems that maturation wins at early age levels, but practice at later ones. It would certainly seem to be clear from reviewing this discussion that learning ability is correlated with age. The older the child becomes, the more important becomes his existing stock of skills, familiarity with symbolic processes, and the like, in undertaking new learning. The fact seems to be that for some time after the child is born the nervous system is being completed, and as this system becomes a mechanically perfect instrument for producing responses, new responses emerge. These responses then become available, so to say, for the learning process. Learning takes over, modifies, and integrates the new response units into the pattern required in a particular society. What the child or animal can do is determined by maturation. What it does do is determined partly by what it can do and partly by the social conditions under which it grows.

The speech of the child naturally attracted the attention of researchers, since man has always been anxious to dilate upon the differences between himself and fellow animals. Through various counts of words and sentences, the vocabulary has been studied at different age levels. A good many vocabulary protocols on initial attempts at speech have been produced. Despite this able and industrious research we still know little about the most important question, namely, how children learn to talk at all, or why they learn to talk. The answer to this question has not been discovered because there has been no context for it. Learning to talk was taken to be somehow "natural" and inevitable, as in most cases it is. Since little was known about the laws of learning in general they could not be applied to this most important area. As knowledge of learning principles has accumulated, the fact that children somehow learn to talk has become more rather than less mysterious. Presently we shall have to devote careful research to this question.

Parallel to the field of language growth, and yet more mysterious, is the growth of emotional habit in children. Clinical reports seem to show that adults continue to exhibit many of the traits acquired in the earliest years of life; at least if one follows the memories of a given adult backward in time he will find reference to many of the traits which the person now shows. These same traits will appear to have a history which is lost beyond the curtain of the individual's earliest memories. It seems likely that fears and inhibitions, acquired drives and dependencies, are learned in the earliest years of life in the interaction between parent and child. Just this learning of intimate emotional habits seems important, since these habits and drives constitute the individual as we intimately know him. This study, already launched and greatly developed through the work of Freud, must receive yet more and closer attention in the research of the future.

Despite all these elements of fact and perspective which the past has provided, I think we must say that we still have no science of child rearing. We have had much brilliant work which has set us on the way. We are beginning to know what are the problems which must be solved by research. Incidentally, I do not say that we "ought" to have a science of child rearing, only that at the moment we do not. It is appropriate now to look ahead and see what landmarks may guide us forward.

Ultimately, the market for a science of child rearing is the parent, and especially the new parent. Discreet bits of excellent research, such as now exist, cannot be very serviceable to the parent. What he needs is a body of theory which covers just those circumstances to which he is exposed, namely, how to treat the child at this and that juncture in its growth so that some desired result in the child's character may be attained. A science of child rearing would provide a theory enabling the prediction of outcomes of different types of training at different ages. Does scheduled feeding, for instance, create such drives within the child as to set up bad emotional habits? Is the fact that the child can be led or forced to accept a feeding schedule germane to the discussion at all? When should cleanliness training be undertaken to get what results in child character? Under what circumstances may or must the parent physically punish the child's responses? How should parents react to the child's aggression, providing always that they can react as they are supposed to? How should taboos on the naïve sex responses of the child be imposed? Does anxiety attached to the child's innocent masturbation generalize to the sex drive and thus operate as a factor in the later sexual life of the person? If anxiety is aroused, does it constitute a frustrating circumstance which, in turn, produces aggression? Is the cross-sex preference of the child a result of training or is it somehow instinctive? How can firm psychosexual attitudes which correspond with the bodily form of the child be engendered?

This seems like a raging mass of questions, and yet they are the very questions on which parents of our day are impaled. Advice

Do We Have a Science of Child Rearing?

on these important matters is now in the realm of hunch, fad, wisdom, guess, or clinical reconstruction. It should be possible to have a science of childhood which is nearer to fact. The theory should be consistent, as our present hunches are not consistent.

For example, many parents are advised today to give the child a kind of freedom which was not permitted in an earlier time, but they are not advised as to what necessary limits to put on this freedom. They must discover for themselves that small children cannot be allowed to play with matches, to manipulate the levers on the gas stove, to run with pointed instruments in the mouth, to move toward the traffic-laden streets, to use the carving knife as a plaything. These parents suffer at having to impose taboos on such actions because they are not told that such limitations are in the interest of the child and are necessary and inevitable. The parent, therefore, suffers from a bad conscience for doing what is his mortal duty.

Perhaps it is a good thing to remove some of the taboos on childhood aggression, but I have seen parents struggling with the following dilemma. A child of four, blessed with the aforementioned freedom from parental restraint, had taken to bashing his one-year-old brother over the head with any handy metal object. The parents were embarrassed at the scenes created but tried to overlook the matter lest the four-year-old should suffer a paralyzing inhibition. At what risk for the future I do not know, these parents were not told that the removal of the taboo on aggression did not include allowing the older child to commit mayhem on his younger brother. They were asked rather, how much serious risk to the younger child they were willing to incur in order to follow their nonaggression pact. Naturally, I have discussed this incident in a one-sided and partisan manner. The parents were also told that they should study the situation and find out and alter, if possible, the factors that were producing such a degree of aggression in the older child. What I want to emphasize is that thanks to the lack of a science of child rearing the parents had received one bit of scientific lore which came inevitably into conflict with another necessity in the same situation.

Where scientists must give such incomplete or contradictory advice we have, of course, no science.

That we have no science of child rearing is not due to the stupidity of child researchers of the past. The emergence of any science is in part a matter of luck. Until all the building blocks necessary for a theory have been assembled, it is difficult to give a consistent account of any natural process. It has been hard to have a science of child rearing without having an adequate theory of how human beings learn. Childhood is notoriously the time of intensive learning. How, then, could we build a science without learning theory?

The new variable of learning theory may indeed liberate child research in new directions and with a new force. As now assembled, learning theory stems from the great tradition in psychology—from Pavlov, Watson, Thorndike, Guthrie, Tolman, Hull, and the work and experiments of hundreds of others. At the Institute of Human Relations at Yale University this theory has received a strong impetus from Freudian theory. In the thought of early behaviorists there was a bias for identifying only the outside stimulus which became connected with a response. Freud's influence has been to identify and stress the importance of "inside" stimuli, of the drive stimuli which are so basic in the understanding of human behavior. This motivational emphasis, borrowed from Freud, has proved easy to naturalize in the field of behavior thinking.

Learning theory now implies that the fundamental variables of drive, response, cue, and reward are among the instruments with which the problem of child development must be attacked. I cannot elaborate them here, but these variables together with other principles and their necessary complications have given us a view of a psychology at once potent enough and flexible enough to deal with human behavior as we intuitively know it. The innate response hierarchy of the child is worked over by the conditions of social life, and in this working over the child's personality is produced.

I have already hinted at the questions which should guide the student of child learning. We need a better analysis of the tasks of childhood. We need to know the response units into which these tasks are broken up so that we can impose such tasks in an orderly manner and in a graded series. Until we have such knowledge we will never be free of the suspicion that we occasionally, and sometimes perhaps continuously over generations, attempt to impose insoluble tasks on our children. Possibly the conditions of cleanliness training, for instance, cannot be altered at the whim of adults or by any psychological fad. It may have its own laws both as to maturation and learning which are tinkered with only at the risk of producing confusion and trauma in the child.

We shall have to learn how language is acquired, since language units apparently function as thought units, and it may well be that the laws of mental life are, in part, those of language acquisition. Possibly in the same inquiry new perspectives on the nature of intelligence will emerge. We know little as yet about the effect of strong drive on the weak ego of very small children. It may be that hunger is an entirely different affair to the newborn child from what it is to the sophisticated adult. Hunger may have a savage and total impact and capacity to create alarm in the infant which have been long since lost to the adult character. Should anything like this be true, our view of the significance of deprivation, even simple-seeming deprivations, to the infant might be radically changed. I can only say that a few clinical experiences of my own have led me to refer to this very earliest period of life as a transitory period of psychosis, that is, a period of strong drive, great helplessness, and weak capacity to react to different real cues in the environment.

Our science-of-childhood-to-be should help us clearly to formulate the alternatives in child learning. We should, indeed, come to think, not of "child training," but rather of child learning. This science should also produce child specialists who can analyze behavior in just the detail here suggested, who have fewer general panaceas and many more detailed investigations of what the child has already learned and what is blocking further learning. The conditions-principles distinction should have great power in this field. Child rearing practice will turn out to be a choice of conditions which are selected to produce particular effects. The principles of learning would seem to be more or less immutable. Conditions are fortunately highly flexible and can be utilized to produce widely varying types of human being.

A word about the techniques of research in child rearing: New scales will have to be invented. Anxiety, for instance, will have to be measured and its relation to other responses determined. Probably a whole host of new measuring instruments will have to be employed to build the science of child rearing. We should, therefore, have scientists at this work who know techniques of scale-making, of pioneering a scale, of testing it for reliability, of testing it for covariance with other scales. The researcher cannot expect that the instruments of other sciences will necessarily enable him to get ahead in this one. It might even be expedient if many of the instruments now in the hands of researchers could be knocked from their hands and they be prevented from measuring the nearest thing measurable in child behavior, letting them "soak" for a while in the problems of childhood, and requiring them to invent appropriate scales to measure the important variables. I do not decry the potential importance of any small bit of fact, but I do much doubt that a science is necessarily created by the accumulation of incidental measurements, however small the error thereof.

Another thing is crucial in regard to a science of child rearing. We may have to abandon the office, the clinic, the white coat, the convenient hours of our present research settings. If we are to study child learning we must study the child where he is learning, and children would seem to learn but precious little in the clinics. We must go to the home with the parents *in situ,* with their particular personalities, and watch their environing effects on the child. This house and these people set up the learning conditions for the child, and we cannot understand what the child learns and why he learns until we see him in relation to his actual home life.

The behavior of children is often mysterious because we do not understand the social conditions which are producing it. I believe child science, once achieved, will have the same magnificent simplicity that is shown by the physical sciences once they

Do We Have a Science of Child Rearing? 49

are achieved. In the absence of knowledge of the appropriate conditions of learning most human behavior is mysterious. We can sweat the mystery out of it by studying the conditions under which it is created.

In this connection I should like to use an analogy which arises in experimental work. Studying the behavior disorder of a child in a clinic is very much like the following fantastic situation. Suppose that after experimenters got through with their experimental rats all those rats were sent to a "rat reject center" and properly mixed up. If a sample of rats was daily withdrawn from this great pool and studied, it would be observed that some would dash down a lighted alley (though rats ordinarily seek the dark). Others would quake to a buzzer. Some would show great ingenuity in escaping from boxes with white walls. Others would jump to almost any sound stimulus. Obviously, little sense could be made out of the behavior of samples of such animals. However, if any of them were seen in the original experimental situation in which they were trained, the behavior would excite no comment. Naturally, the rat rushes down the lighted alley where it has been fed. It seeks to escape the stimuli of white walls where it has been shocked.

So also I presume it to be with children. If a child is dependent we should seek the circumstances under which such a mighty dependence was demanded of him. If he is aggressive we should learn why these behavior patterns helped the child to meet his life needs. If the child lies we should search out the circumstances, probably inadvertently set up, which have rewarded lying.

Never was the prayer for a great philanthropist to sponsor a radical departure in child research more fervently uttered than now. Research in the home is a time-taking task even if only behavior samples are taken. The work is probably sex specialized and must be carried on by women, since most men will not allow other men to browse around their households even under the noblest of pretexts. Possibly the research operator should also have a conventional role in the household and possibly also should perform some helpful tasks. In this connection I have thought of the registered nurse. With some additional scientific training added to the curriculum of the modern university school of nursing, the nurse might have exactly the combination of qualities and talents needed. Once the fundamental situation was established by the nurse, male researchers could presumably work with her from time to time and could certainly aid in the design of the research situation, the invention of the necessary scales, and the analysis of the data.

The urgency of developing a science of child rearing is emphasized by the many faddish innovations in our traditional child culture which have arisen from the partial sciences of the present day. With each new idea, fad, or tendency in science new recommendations have been made to parents. There has been a rapid turnover of such fads, but short-lived as they are, they have served to disrupt the traditional units of our child rearing techniques. It may well be that while our child rearing has gained something in flexibility it has lost much in unity and consistency since the days of our great-grandmothers, and it may also be that far from being ahead, we have a piecemeal, patchwork kind of child science which is actually less adaptive than the uninfluenced techniques of earlier times.

For example, Watson emphasized the importance of habit in human behavior. As a result, parents were asked whether or not they stood for "habit" in the training of their children. They answered, of course, that they did, and were given a good deal of advice on "regularity," "system," and organization which, for all we know, has been very bad for children. We now know, as scientists, that Watson's doctrine on habit omitted the crucial emotional elements of drive and reward and that inferences made from it in regard to the behavior of children were bound to be similarly biased. There must be times when bad science is worse than no science at all. Researchers must certainly be exceedingly careful not to give advice beyond the specific implications of their data.

Similarly, Adler's emphasis on the dangers of childish selfishness and the tendency to dominate has resulted in a ludicrous, counteractive attitude. Parents have come to fear that early in-

Do We Have a Science of Child Rearing?

dulgence will create dependence and have inferred that the earlier the child is taught the bitter way of the world the better it will be for the child. In some circles this amounts almost to regarding the newborn child as a kind of enemy who must be rapidly put in his place before he dominates the family entirely. We cannot say that Adler is wrong, but we can certainly offer an alternative point of view (although it may be no better than his) to wit, that the child should be granted the greatest indulgence when it exhibits the greatest helplessness and that the strait jacket of reality should be only slowly tightened around its body.

Similarly but conversely, the Freudian emphasis on the importance of indulgence in early months and years may be incorrectly applied. Some parents have extended the indulgence to later years when, not indulgence, but proportionate enforcement of cultural demands is required. If the child is to be made responsible and capable he must know at one and the same time that he will get what he needs when need is desperate but that under most circumstances he must work and bear and renounce in order to live in the world as it is. When upon the base laid down by Freud, a real science of childhood is built, it will be impossible for such confusing interpretations to be made and for irresponsible interpretations of research to get abroad. The great importance of science, as compared with a series of isolated observations, is that it can give a proportionate and consistent set of rules and study the alternatives in case this or that practice is followed. Since a science must deal with all the problems in a particular culture at one time it is less likely to give inconsistent or whimsical advice.

Many now believe that our practices in the field of child rearing are to a great extent related to the later happiness, freedom, and effectiveness of individual personalities. This would render the creation of a child science of highest importance even though there were no other issues at stake. But there are other issues at stake.

It may be that in a time of crisis, such as the present, our child culture may prove to be unexpectedly related to national survival itself. The reactions of childhood which become strong habits are believed to persist into adult life and to be transferred to adult symbols and institutions. Thus the child with a grudge against his parents may become the adult with a grudge against his nation, his social group, his religion, or some other aspect of adult social structure. If this were the case, the creation of a science of child rearing would not be optional but would be felt by all to be an urgent and even desperate need.

For example, in our time there has been a marked growth of antidemocratic ideology. This growth of antidemocratic sentiment is, in part, based upon persisting injustices within the societies called "democratic." In the United States we still suffer the abomination of a caste system. Many of the effects of a highly stratified class society are also with us, damaging the self-esteem and sense of worth of many citizens. These circumstances have promoted and seem to justify a degree of hostility toward our society which has, of course, taken the familiar form of suggestions for social change. If we may judge by the situation in the world today these suggestions have not been acted upon with sufficient rapidity, and many people sense a great disparity between the conditions they are forced to bear and the possible social conditions which might now easily exist for them. In the United States we have means and techniques for producing social change, though some of our greatest changes seem to be coincidental with other great activities like the conduct of a war. Nevertheless, the movement toward a square-deal society is clear today, though sometimes it seems to be unbearably slow. If our people are patient under this slowness it is possibly because "standing in line" is an American tradition along with dreaming of being at the ticket window.

However, by no means all the hostility toward our current society depends upon real, adult deprivations. Many hate our society for the "wrongs" done them in childhood, the stupidities of hunger and neglect all the more damnable because avoidable. A doctrine like that of Karl Marx acts to release these hatreds, to liberate the conscience to hate in the name of defending the weak, the helpless, and the exploited.

Many find our sexual mores hard to bear and develop a certain hostility toward society on the ground of frustration in this

Do We Have a Science of Child Rearing? 53

sphere. They have experienced the confusion and hardly tolerable privation produced by our sex training and have lived to be vaguely miserable adults, chronically resentful of they know not what. There is in them, nevertheless, a persisting hope for sexual liberation, a liberation which would seem possible within our present moral order, the goal of which might be conventionally expressed as the creation of husbands and wives who can make use of their sexual opportunities within marriage, to make the difficult married state bearable or even desirable.

I have often thought that the malcontents of our time do not so much want a better society as, really, no society at all, and therefore they wish to destroy our own. I think in this connection of the American physicist who at a public conference hoped that "others" would measure and publish the constants necessary to control the release of atomic energy. He thought it shameful that these were in American hands only and was apparently giving broad hints to fellow physicists in foreign lands who might be overhearing him. I for one felt that this man knew too much and that he expressed a petulant and dangerous impatience with "democratic" processes which seemed unreasonable and not intelligible on any rational ground.

The way before us is clear enough. The avoidable differences and discriminations must be avoided. The caste system must be abolished; anxieties about sheer physical survival must be ended. Status inequalities must be equalized, and where they do exist they must be placed on the basis of service, work, and talent. But these changes do not mean revolution and need not be achieved by revolutionary means. I believe that if democracy can intolerantly and ruthlessly demand the necessary time it can work itself over into a more satisfactory system. Anyone who pushes too hard in the line will have to be shown his place by the policeman. The line forms to the right and coils up and ever up the hill. That is the way, I take it, that we dream of working out our social salvation. If there are some ahead of us we will let them have their turn for the time being so long as the line does not form in the same order before every booth. That kind of line is gone forever.

Let me suppose for the moment that we know now what we are

going to know in a hundred more years about a science of child rearing. What use would we make of our knowledge? Suppose that we could make our children more peaceable than present-day children, less dependent than present-day children, less inhibited than present-day children, less aggressive than present-day children, more reflective and planful than our children are now, would we dare do it, and if so, what parts of it?

It is hard to know. Certainly we do not wish to modify our child culture to the extent of national extinction. Possibly, for the world we now face, we should strive for yet more aggressive children. Perhaps they will be needed as adults if our society is to survive and have a chance to evolve. Possibly, in order even to try our own scheme, we must be ready to stamp out those who would move faster by violent means.

Perhaps, on the other hand, creating greater hostility might recoil on us. Hostile adults might take their own society as the target and thus be the death of us. Perhaps the correct move would be to make our children love their parents and our society more than they do now. For the supreme aggressions, should they be necessary, can occur only in the name of love.

This way of thought is dark indeed. Without knowledge of the kind of world the child will find when he becomes an adult we cannot choose the type of personality we will seek to develop. Even if we had a science of child rearing we could not use it in the absence of the ground plan of a specific adult society for which the child is being prepared. We might use our child science considerably to cut down individual misery in any particular society but we would always do this at the risk of changing characteristics which might be necessary for social survival.

Even though we were to let matters alone until social forces at the adult level had had a chance to shake down into a more stable order we would still be urgently impelled to create the science on the basis of which personality could be formed, for there is probably no form of overhead social system which can permanently maintain itself as a world-wide society if men are made intrinsically hostile and bellicose from their earliest experiences in life. Sooner or later the mischief-makers, the seekers after chaos, will creep into the control apparatus of the society and work their destruction there. If we are to build and maintain a peaceable society we must train men from earliest life in the habits of a peaceable society. This means creating the conditions from earliest life which will reward justice, sharing, bearing, waiting, foresight, and planning.

The vista has been opened to us of the creation of human personality and of a world order to match. The two supreme achievements awaiting the mind of man lie down the road. We know this road to be that of science. We do not expect that a peaceable society will necessarily be an idyllic one nor that a maximally healthy personality can exist without conflict and misery. Man in his social and personal life is bound to show the effects of his thousands of generations of struggle and passion. His intemperate nature will therefore leave its marks on his society and on his person. Common sense and mother wit have nevertheless advanced him a long way toward control of his environment and himself. In the more refined form of reasoning and foresight, with the aid of scientific control and caution, we believe that he can create a more bearable personal and social life. In the name of good men everywhere I propose that we get on with the task.

Child Rearing in the Class Structure of American Society

W. ALLISON DAVIS

THE STUDY OF AMERICAN SOCIAL CLASSES has become a very complex field. This approach to the comparative, or differential, psychology of our social strata has been used in the study of American moral controls, familial organization and mores, child rearing, adolescent personality, projective responses, sex behavior, illness, politics, rackets, industrial conflict, the public educational system, the courts, the churches, the organizations, the processes involved in rising in the world, or falling in the world, and in still other major areas of behavior. In the study of basic socialization, the social-class approach in recent years has been developed systematically by John Dollard and others in the attempt to understand the processes by which human beings learn their social drives, their morals, their emotional values, and by Harold Jones in respect to intelligence.

All students in this field realize, however, that they have been able to drop too few sounding lines into the "lower depths" of the class system, into the bottom one third of the American population. This is still the no-man's land of social psychology. Our attempt here is to place the observational hints and the limited quantitative data we have about slum culture into a few basic hypotheses about the cultural motivation, or social learning, of slum groups.

Social classes essentially operate so as to maintain barriers against intimate social participation. Those individuals, families, and social cliques which refer to each other in popular language as "nice" or "respectable" seldom have any intimate association,

Child Rearing in American Society

either at work or in their homes, with any people from those families which are vulgarly called "common," "ignorant," or "low." To put it more graphically, most people from the "wrong side of the tracks" have no intimate association in any form, as equals, with people from the "right side of the tracks." People of the slums are barred from social participation both with the Gold Coast and "respectable," middle-class Suburbia. Indeed, they are also stigmatized and avoided by the small "respectable" people (the lower middle class) who may live in the same block. Finally, the "bottom third" is likewise avoided by "the poor, but honest and clean" families, as they think of themselves, that is, the top part of the working class.

People cannot learn their mores, social drives, values—their basic culture—from books. One can learn a particular culture and a particular moral system only from those people who know and exhibit this behavior in frequent relationships with the learner. If a child can associate intimately with no one but slum adults and children, he can learn only slum culture. The pivotal meaning of social classes to the student of behavior, therefore, is that they limit and systematize the learning environment of their members. Thus each class has developed its own characteristic and adaptive form of the American basic culture. Each member of a social class learns this cultural behavior from his family, his gang or play group, his social clique, and his other intimate groups.

Generally, culture includes all behavior which men learn in conformity with a group of people. In the slum, as elsewhere, the human group evolves solutions to the basic problems of group life, that is, the problems of subsistence, of unity of the kinship group, sex control, child rearing, direction of, and defense against, aggression, relation to the supernatural, social recreation, and so on. Because the slum individual usually is responding to a different physical, economic, and cultural reality from that in which the middle-class individual is trained, the slum individual's habits and values also must be different, if they are to be realistic. The behavior which we regard as "delinquent" or "shiftless" or "unmotivated" in slum groups is usually a perfectly realistic, adaptive, and, in slum life, respectable response to reality.

By defining the people with whom an individual may have intimate social relationships, therefore, our social class system narrows his learning and training environment. His social instigations and goals, his symbolic world and its evaluation, are largely selected from the narrow culture of that class with which alone he can associate freely.

A child's social learning takes place chiefly in the environment of his family, his family's social clique, and his own social clique. The instigations, goals, and controls both of the family and of the intimate clique are a function principally of their class ways, that is, of the status demands in their part of the society. The number of class controls and dogmas which a child must learn and struggle continually to maintain, in order to meet his family's status demands as a class unit, is very great. Class training of the child ranges all the way from the control of the times and ritual by which he eats his food to the control of his choice of playmates and of his educational and occupational goals.

Our knowledge of social class training is now sufficient to enable us to say that no studies can henceforth generalize about "the child." We shall always have to ask, "A child of what social class, in what environment?" Very few statements which one might make concerning the physical growth, the socialization, or the motivation of slum children, for example, would hold for upper middle-class children.

Class ways in child training, as well as the class-motivating factors in the child's social learning, differ sharply even when the observer considers only the classes having low status. The social drives and goals of the lower middle class, for example, are fundamentally unlike those of the lower class. In education and social work today, the ineffectiveness of middle-class values upon the great masses of lower-class children and adults probably is the crucial dilemma of our thoroughly middle-class teaching and social work staffs. The processes underlying our failure are not yet entirely clear. It seems probable from life histories, however, that lower-class children remain unsocialized and unmotivated

Child Rearing in American Society

(from the viewpoint of middle-class culture) because (1) they are humiliated and punished too severely by teachers for having the lower-class culture which their own mothers, fathers, and friends approve; and (2) because emotional and social rewards are systematically denied to the lower-class child and adult by the systems of privilege existing in the school and in the larger society.

To understand the socialization of slum children, one must first view the slum adult world, and trace the motivational system which slum adults exhibit as a group. What are the basic social drives of slum adults? To put this question more carefully, what experiences does the slum individual learn from his group to define as "pleasant" or as "painful" among the available experiences in his world?

This approach seems to be the quickest route to an understanding of the social motivation of any group; for we know from anthropologists that the primary function of all cultures is to teach the members of the group to regard certain experiences as pleasant and others as painful. That is to say, nearly all "rewards" and "punishments," so-called, vary with regard to their particular form, intensity, and meaning from culture to culture. We wish to know, therefore (1) what experiences seem, to the slum group, to be most attainable, pleasant, and free from anxiety; and (2) what experiences seem most unpleasant, or most dangerous to the physical survival or social acceptance of the individual. Anyone who has tried to increase the motivation of slum individuals to work regularly knows that these are not simple questions.

Experiences defined by slum culture as unpleasant.—One of the most basic differences in motivation between lower-class and middle-class people is their attitude toward eating. Owing to the greater security of their food supply, middle-class people eat more regularly. They therefore have learned to eat more sparingly at any given time, because they know that they are certain of their next meal. They have also developed a conscientious taboo upon "overeating"; they feel some guilt about getting fat and about what they call "raiding the icebox."

Slum people, however, have an uncertain food supply. The fear that they will not get enough to eat develops soon after the nursing period. Therefore, when the supply is plentiful, they eat as much as they can hold. They "pack food away" in themselves as a protection against the shortage which will develop before the next payday. They wish to get fat, for they regard fat as a protection against tuberculosis and physical weakness. Basically, the origin of this attitude toward eating is their deep fear of starvation.

Just as food anxiety is far more urgent in lower-class than it is in middle-class society, so is the anxiety which is aroused by the danger of eviction from shelter, the danger of having too little sleep, the danger of being cold, and the danger of being in the dark. The middle-class individual is relatively certain that he will have enough coal or light; he buys his coal by the ton or the five tons; he burns five or ten electric lights. The lower-class person's hold upon fire for heating is on a day-to-day or week-to-week basis. He buys coal by the bushel, or the five bushels, or by one-ton loads. Every week or so, therefore, he has to face the fear of being cold, and of having his children cold.

Similarly with light, his anxiety is chronic and realistic. His evenings are spent in a gray light; if more than one or two bulbs are used, and if those are not of the lowest candle power, he will not be able to pay the light bill. Therefore, the fear of not having so basic a necessity as light—a fear which middle-class people escape after childhood—is recurrent with the slum individual. Walk into any slum neighborhood at night. People are crowded together in a dingy, twilight world. Their streets and alleys likewise are full of darkness, so that their chronic expectation of assault or rape is increased.

Just as slum people have painful, anxiety-ridden associations with food, so they have with shelter, sleep, and darkness. To this list must be added the fear of being inadequately clothed in winter. Most slum men, Negroes and whites, have no overcoat in normal times. Most sharecroppers' children have no woolen clothes in cold, winter weather.

Now, when these same people get relatively large increases in income—as they did during the war—they spend their money "extravagantly," as middle-class people judge their behavior.

What is the meaning of this "plunging" for fur coats, for expensive clothes for children, for new furniture? Part of the motivation is a drive for prestige symbols, an attempt to acquire some of the signs of middle-class status. Equally important in the pattern, certainly, is its function as a defense against anxiety, which is similar to their Gargantuan eating after payday. When a person in this class has money, he buys things which he will be able to buy only once or twice in his lifetime, such as respectable or warm clothes and a "decent" bed. He burns all the light he wants; he eats great quantities of meat.

Thus, lower-class people look upon life as a recurrent series of depressions and peaks with regard to the gratification of their basic needs. In their lives it is all or nothing, or next-to-nothing. When they have fire, their homes are stifling hot, and everyone sits as close to the fire as possible; for they remember anxiously what it was to be cold, to be too cold to sit in the house, so cold that the whole family must go to bed to keep warm. Just as their deep anxiety about starvation leads them, even in "good times," to glut themselves, as middle-class people view their eating, so does the learned fear of deprivation drive lower-class people to get all they can of the other physical gratifications "while the getting is good."

It would be more rational if they saved and budgeted their money, but human beings are not rational. They are what their culture teaches them to be. "Man is a reasoning, but not a reasonable animal." Lower-class people cannot learn middle-class foresight and moderation unless they can participate socially with middle-class people, whom they may then learn to imitate. So far, the public school is our only chance to teach lower-class people the middle-class motivational pattern. But the schools do not yet understand how to reward lower-class pupils. Furthermore, our economic system does not offer any prospect of a regular income to slum people; therefore, they lack the relative security which must underlie habits of saving, buying insurance, purchasing homes, etc. As the average slum worker says, "Why should I try to save? The little bit I could put aside will be gone six months after the next depression starts."

Turning now to those experiences which are defined as painful chiefly by the social, as contrasted with the physical, environment, we find that the socially based anxieties are still more numerous. The middle-class view that slum people have no sense of respectability, feel no pressure for social conformity, is simply ignorance of the facts. Lower-class culture includes a vast number of social taboos, and therefore stimulates a great number of social anxieties. First, to return to the so-called "physical" area of food, shelter, and heat, slum culture has its own "decent" or "respectable" standards for food and housing. Lower-class people learn their own group's cultural standard of "enough to eat," or "a good house," or "good furniture." It is probable that only when the cultural goals for subsistence (as "subsistence" is defined by slum culture) are threatened, therefore, does the person experience marked anxiety. Lower-class people consider as "good" the same house or job which middle-class people regard as humiliating. The same standard of living that raises the anxiety of middle-class people will greatly allay the anxiety of slum people, in our present social system.

The socially defined dangers of slum life originate in the threat of disapproval, ridicule, or rejection of the individual by his family, play group, gang, church, club, and so on. All these lower-class groups make cultural demands of the child and adolescent, just as do the middle-class family, play group, and club. But the demands are generally different from those of the middle-class group. In other words, the lower-class individual is taught by his culture to be anxious about different social dangers.

Whereas the middle-class child learns a socially adaptive fear of receiving poor grades in school, of being aggressive toward the teacher, of fighting, of cursing, and of having early sex relations, the slum child learns to fear quite different social acts. His gang teaches him to fear being "taken in" by the teacher, of being a "softie" with her. To study "homework" seriously is literally a disgrace. Instead of boasting of good marks in school, one conceals them, if one ever receives any. The lower-class adolescent fears not to be thought a street-fighter; it is a suspicious and dangerous social trait. He fears not to curse. If he cannot claim early sex relations, his virility is seriously questioned.

Thus society raises many anxieties in slum people also, but with regard to the attainment of goals which seem strange to middle-class people. For those who must live in a slum community, however, these goals are realistic and adaptive.

Experiences defined by slum culture as pleasant.—There is space here to consider only two areas of experience which are patterned by slum culture as chiefly pleasant. I do not believe that there is any evidence that these two areas, sex relations and physical aggression, are more basic physiologically than the food area, or the heat-cold area, of experience. Psychologically, however, the areas of sex and aggression are the most formative of middle-class personality, because middle-class culture teaches the individual, from childhood, that sexual responses and physical aggression, more than any other behaviors, must be either inhibited or very carefully controlled.

The result of this middle-class training of children to fear their own sex impulses and their rage is usually to make sex and aggression the chief problem areas of the middle-class personality. The manifestations of these two types of problem are usually highly disguised, but the source is very simple. Sex and aggression (including stealing) become, if not "properly" controlled and guided according to the middle-class cultural standard, the most dangerous forms of behavior to a person of middle-class status. The middle-class child is taught this lesson by precept and example. For a large proportion of middle-class people, therefore, sex has been stamped as "dirty," or "unimportant," and filled with anxiety, because both in childhood and adolescence their own sexual responses were made to appear too dangerous socially by their parents and teachers.

In slum groups, on the other hand, both children and adults are permitted far more gratification of their sexual responses and of their rage responses. This permissiveness, as it seems to middle-class people, extends into most of the other basic areas of child rearing in the lower class. I shall deal briefly, therefore, with the training and cultural motivation of the lower-class child and adolescent, in respect to the basic types of gratification.

In a recent study of child rearing practices in 100 white and 100 Negro middle-class and lower-class families in Chicago, Dr. Robert J. Havighurst and I discovered:

1. That more lower-class than middle-class babies are breast-fed only
2. That more lower-class babies are fed at will
3. That more lower-class than middle-class white babies have the breast or bottle longer than twelve months
4. That lower-class children are weaned later
5. That bowel training is begun earlier, on the average, with middle-class children
6. That bladder training is begun earlier, on the average, with middle-class children
7. That middle-class children are expected to help at home earlier
8. That middle-class children are expected to assume responsibility earlier
9. That lower-class children stay up later, stay in the streets later, and go to the movies more often

All these differences between social classes, with regard to child rearing, were statistically significant.

This study of white and Negro families in Chicago confirms previous exploratory observational studies. It seems clear, therefore, that, as compared with the rearing of middle-class children, the early training environment of most lower-class children permits them fuller gratification of their organically based drives. The cultural training of the eating, eliminating, and exploring drives is applied much more gradually, and relapses are treated far more leniently. Yet, according to their mothers, lower-class children succeed in learning their toilet habits by exactly the same median age as do the early-pressed middle-class children. The one exception to this rule is that of the bowel training of Negro children. Middle-class Negro children complete this training much earlier (at thirteen months) than do lower-class Negro children (eighteen months) or white children of either social class (eighteen months). In many respects, we know, the Negro middle class is a very conservative group.

The findings concerning thumb-sucking seem to support the theory that the middle-class child experiences in his cultural training a more depriving attack upon his sources of organic and emotional support than does the lower-class child; for three times as many white middle-class children as white lower-class children were reported to suck their thumbs. We would expect this higher incidence of thumb-sucking among middle-class children, in line with the theory that thumb-sucking is a response to strong interference with the hunger drive, and with the pleasure drive in sucking. Yet Negro middle-class children, who were trained much more permissively than white middle-class children with respect to nursing and weaning, but much more rigorously than white middle-class children with respect to toilet habits, sucked their thumbs in almost the same proportion as that reported for the white middle-class. We conclude, therefore, that thumb-sucking, like nail-biting and nose-picking, may be a response to frustration of any sort rather than to frustration in the feeding and sucking areas only.

Masturbation seems to admit of the same interpretation. We know that the average middle-class parent is more watchful and punitive than the average lower-class parent in dealing with genital play. In spite of this supervision, three times as many white middle-class as lower-class children were reported to masturbate. Among Negroes, twice as many middle-class as lower-class children were reported as masturbating. Thus it appears that masturbation in children may not be primarily a response to a direct sexual drive, but rather a response to any or all of several kinds of frustration, each of which is more common in the rigorous training of middle-class children.

It seems true, then, that middle-class children are early taught to accept greater restraint, and to become more tame with regard to the direct use of their own sources of primary organic satisfaction.

Before comparing middle-class and lower-class adolescents, a warning must be injected. We recall that the long, indulgent nursing period of lower-class infants does not prevent their developing marked fear of starvation in later childhood and adulthood. This fact means that new situations, if strongly organized physically or socially, make new behavior. This is a cardinal principle of the new integrated science of social psychology. Basic learning can and does appear at any age level, provided that society or the physical environment changes the organization of its basic rewards and punishments for the individual.

Secondly, we should not be so naïve as to think that lower-class life is a happy hunting ground, given over to complete impulse expression. Slum people must accept all the basic sexual controls on incest, on homosexuality, on having more than one mate at a time, and on marital irresponsibility. In fact, there is evidence to indicate that slum people are more observant of the taboos upon incest and homosexuality than are those in the upper class. Furthermore, the same pattern which holds in their food intake—deprivation, relieved by peaks of great indulgence—is typical of lower-class sexual life. Lack of housing, lack of a bed for oneself, frequent separations of mates or lovers, the hard daily work of mothers with six to fourteen children, the itinerant life of the men, all make sexual life less regular, secure, and routine than in the middle class. In the slum, one certainly does not have a sexual partner for as many days each month as do middle-class married people, but one gets and gives more satisfaction, over longer periods, when one does have a sexual partner. With this reservation in mind, we may proceed to examine adolescent behavior in the two classes.

The aggressive behavior of adolescents is a crucial case in point. In the middle class, aggression is clothed in the conventional forms of "initiative," or "ambition," or even of "progressiveness," but in the lower class it more often appears unabashed as physical attack, or as threats of, and encouragement for, physical attack. In general, middle-class aggression is taught to adolescents in the form of social and economic skills which will enable them to compete effectively at that level. The lower classes not uncommonly teach their children and adolescents to strike out with fist or knife and to be certain to hit first. Both girls and boys at ado-

Child Rearing in American Society

lescence may curse their father to his face or even attack him with fists, sticks, or axes in free-for-all family encounters. Husbands and wives sometimes stage pitched battles in the home; wives have their husbands arrested; and husbands, when locked out, try to break in or burn down their own homes. Such fights with fists or weapons, and the whipping of wives, occur sooner or later in most lower-class families. They may not appear today, nor tomorrow, but they will appear if the observer remains long enough.

The important consideration with regard to physical aggression in lower-class adolescents is, therefore, that it is learned as an approved and socially rewarded form of behavior in their culture. An interviewer recently observed two nursery school boys from lower-class families; they were boasting about the length of their fathers' clasp knives! The parents themselves have taught their children to fight, not only children of either sex, but also adults who "make trouble" for them. If the child or adolescent cannot whip a grown opponent, his father or mother will join the fight. In such lower-class groups, an adolescent boy who does not try to be a good fighter will not receive the approval of his father, nor will he be acceptable to any play group or gang. The result of these cultural sanctions is that he learns to fight and to admire fighters. The conception that aggression and hostility are neurotic or maladaptive symptoms of a chronically frustrated adolescent is an ethnocentric view of middle-class individuals. In lower-class families, physical aggression is as much a normal, socially approved, and socially inculcated type of behavior as it is in frontier communities.

There are many forms of aggression, of course, which are disapproved by lower-class as well as by middle-class adolescents. These include, among others, attack by magic or poison, rape, and cutting a woman in the face. Yet all these forms of aggression are fairly common in some lower-class areas. Stealing is another form of aggression which lower-class parents verbally forbid, but which some of them in fact allow—so long as their child does not steal from his family or its close friends. The model of the adolescent's play group and of his own kin, however, is the crucial determinant of his behavior. Even where the efforts of the parent to instill middle-class mores in the child are more than half-hearted, the power of the street culture in which the child and adolescent are trained overwhelms the parental verbal instruction. The rewards of gang prestige, freedom of movement, and property gain all seem to be on the side of the street culture.

Like physical aggression, sexual relationships and motivation are more direct and uninhibited in lower-class adolescents. The most striking departure from the usual middle-class motivation is that, in much lower-class life, sexual drives and behavior in children are not regarded as inherently taboo and dangerous.

There are many parents in low-status culture, of course, who taboo these behaviors for their girls. Mothers try to prevent daughters from having children before they are married, but the example of the girl's own family is often to the contrary. At an early age the child learns of common-law marriages and of extra-marital relationships of men and women in his own family. He sees his father disappear to live with other women, or he sees other men visit his mother or married sisters. Although none of his siblings may be illegitimate, the chances are very high that sooner or later his father and mother will accuse each other of having illegitimate children; or that at least one of his brothers or sisters will have a child outside marriage. His play group, girls and boys, discuss sexual relations frankly at the age of eleven or twelve, and he gains status with them by beginning intercourse early.

With sex, as with aggression, therefore, the social instigations and reinforcements of adolescents who live in these different cultures are opposites. The middle-class adolescent is punished for physical aggression and for physical sexual relations; the lower-class adolescent is frequently rewarded, both socially and organically, for these same behaviors. The degree of anxiety, guilt, or frustration attached to these behaviors, therefore, is entirely different in the two cases. One might go so far as to say that in the case of middle-class adolescents such anxiety and guilt, with regard to physical aggression and sexual intercourse, are proof of their normal socialization in their culture. In lower-class adolescents in certain environments, they are evidence of revolt against their own class culture, and possibly of incipient personality difficulties.

The point which these considerations seems to make clear, and which seems to be borne out by many detailed life histories of adolescents of each class, is as follows: The social reality of individuals differs in the most fundamental respects according to their status and culture. The individuals of different class cultures are reacting to different situations. If they are realistic in their responses to these situations, their drives and goals will be different. This basic principle of comparative psychology implies that in order to decide whether an individual in American society is normal or neurotic, one must know his social class and likewise his ethnic culture. He may be quite poorly oriented with regard to middle-class culture, simply because he has not been trained in it and, therefore, does not respond to its situations. If his behavior is normal for lower-class culture—which clinicians, teachers, and guidance workers do not usually know—he may appear to them to be maladjusted, unmotivated, unsocialized, or even neurotic. In dealing with such cases, the reference points of social reality of the teacher or psychologist must be set up with regard to the basic demands of lower-class culture upon its members.

Adolescence in Our Society

HAROLD E. JONES

The period of adolescence is sometimes referred to as a flowering and fulfillment, sometimes as a calamity. Taken literally, adolescence is the process of becoming adult, growing into maturity. But the term has gained other, less favorable meanings. These are implied when we speak of adolescent "stress and strain," "growing pains," "teen-age troubles," "the silly phase," and other phenomena to which we attach the adjective "adolescent," sometimes in a resigned mood and sometimes in exasperation.

Many persons have raised the question of whether this process of growing up is naturally and inevitably a difficult one, or whether its painfulness is in some sense a disease of society, and therefore remediable through appropriate social changes. The answer to this question has varied widely according to the preoccupations of the person answering it. The biological answer stresses changes in hormone secretions, changes in the rate of skeletal growth, and temporary imbalances in body structure and function. It is these imbalances, we are told, which are the immediate source of adolescent maladjustment. The sociological and anthropological answer, on the other hand, stresses the conditions and demands of the culture in which the child is growing up. It is pointed out that the same processes of biological maturing that place a child in jeopardy in one culture may offer no special problems in another culture. Each of these answers is a partial one. Adolescence is not necessarily a period of acute disturbance. When disturbance occurs, the determining agencies lie in multiple form both in the organism and in society; we cannot hope to achieve understanding or control if we look at merely one of these two groups of factors.

It may be appropriate to begin this discussion with some account of the physical aspects of adolescence and of the developmental processes which set off this period so clearly from earlier childhood.

First, we know that at about eight or nine years of age on an average, in girls, and some two years later in boys, a change occurs in the rate of physical growth.[1] In the preceding years, ever since early childhood, growth has occurred at a fairly even and steady pace; growth in height, for example, involves gains of about 4 percent per year during these childhood years. But now, near the end of childhood, growth becomes slower; there is often a pause which marks the transition point between the slow, gradual development of childhood and the accelerated, more irregular growth changes of adolescence. It is as though the organism needed a little time in which to consolidate childhood gains, to muster resources, and to get ready for the abrupt transformations that are now to take place. This is a figurative way of putting it, but it does appear that we have during this period an interval in which the growth controls of childhood are fading and the adolescent growth factors are not yet fully ready to function.

In some respects, the problems of adolescence bear a resemblance to the problems of infancy, so that adolescence is sometimes called a second infancy. Physiologically, this may in a way be justified, in view of the fact that infants show an instability in many physiological processes, and gradually win a greater degree of equilibrium. With the beginning of the puberal cycle we have a renewal of unstable conditions. Basal metabolism, for example, may show marked fluctuations at this time.[2]

In an adult such metabolic changes could readily be a matter of some concern; in an adolescent they are physiological in the sense that they are very commonly and perhaps normally shown in the process of adjusting to the new phase of more rapid growth and to new conditions in the internal environment. At the same

---

[1] Frank K. Shuttleworth, *The Physical and Mental Growth of Girls and Boys, Age Six to Nineteen, in Relation to Age at Maximal Growth* (Washington, D.C.: Society for Research in Child Development, 1939).

[2] Nathan W. Shock, "The Effect of Menarche on Basal Physiological Functions in Girls," *American Journal of Physiology*, CXXXIX, No. 2 (June, 1943), 288–92.

time, changes are also occurring in other basal functions. Among girls, for example, in the three years just preceding the menarche the average pulse rate increases and then decreases; the systolic blood pressure increases and then levels off.[3]

It is not surprising that the adjustments in bodily processes should not always be smooth and orderly. The adolescent awkwardness, which we sometimes observe at the level of motor skills, may have its parallel in a kind of physiological awkwardness. The transition to a changed body economy may be difficult, and there may be further difficulties because of an interacting relationship with social and psychological transitions.

In a standard work on pediatrics the author observes that "the age of puberty is attended with many dangers to health. The changes in the organs are sudden. The heart grows larger, the blood vessels narrower. . . . At this time particularly mental disorders may develop and hereditary defects appear. Anemic conditions arise and may be followed by constitutional diseases. . . ."[4] Such statements may cause unnecessary alarm and overemphasize the health hazards of adolescence, and yet it is true that the morbidity rate increases during the 'teens, and you have only to enter any classroom of adolescent youngsters to observe in posture, skin color, and, particularly, in skin conditions such as acne, abundant evidence of defects in the smooth course of adolescent maturing. Growth discrepancies also occur in the proportionate development of legs, arms, and trunk and in the deposition of fat. The timing of growth for different parts of the body may vary in different individuals, resulting in cases of poorly synchronized and markedly disproportionate development.[5]

Psychoanalysts have emphasized another way in which adolescence is like a second infancy, in that it involves a recurrence, in

[3] Nathan W. Shock, "Basal Blood Pressure and Pulse Rate in Adolescents," *American Journal of Diseases of Children*, LXVIII, No. 1 (July, 1944), 16–22.

[4] John Diven, "Peculiarities of Disease in Childhood," in *Pediatrics*, ed. Abt (Philadelphia: Saunders, 1923), II, 192.

[5] Herbert R. and Lois M. Stolz, "Adolescent Problems Related to Somatic Variations," in *Forty-third Yearbook of the National Society for the Study of Education* (Chicago: Chicago University, Department of Education, 1944), Part I, "Adolescence," pp. 80–89.

their terms, of infantile sexual impulses. The increased sexual drives of adolescence are countered by inhibitions; the adolescent may be afraid of these drives in the genital form in which they now appear, and may regress to more familiar infantile forms of sexuality. Fenichel points out that adolescence is often marked by contradictory psychological expressions: "Egoism and altruism, pettiness and generosity, sociability and loneliness, cheerfulness and sadness, silly jocularity and overseriousness, intense loves and sudden abandonment of these loves, submission and rebellion, materialism and idealism, rudeness and tender consideration—all are typical." [6] These contradictions as cited by Fenichel are related to the fact that in adolescence there appear side by side or following one another "genital heterosexual impulses, all kinds of infantile sexual behavior, and attitudes of extreme asceticism, which not only try to repress all sexuality but everything pleasant as well." [7] The intensification of the sexual impulses at puberty, and the resulting conflicts, mark the end of the relatively peaceful latency period. Fenichel expresses the view that all the mental phenomena characteristic of puberty may be regarded as reactions to these disturbances, and as attempts to re-establish the equilibrium of the latency period, and he adds that "in a society that treated infantile sexuality differently puberty, too, would assume a different course." [8]

In commenting upon this interpretation we may return again to our earlier statement that the difficulties of adolescence have a multiple origin and cannot be interpreted solely in terms of psychological, or cultural, or biological agencies. The student of child development is aware of many factors, by no means evidently related to sexual dilemmas or the Oedipus complex, which emerge at puberty to bedevil and perplex the child, his parents, and his teachers. Some of these factors have already been mentioned in connection with disturbances in physiological functions and in physical growth. Since adolescence is a period of increased susceptibility to psychosomatic disorders, no doubt a

---

[6] Otto Fenichel, *The Psychoanalytic Theory of Neurosis* (New York: Norton, 1945), p. 111.
[7] *Ibid.*, pp. 110–11.   [8] *Ibid.*, p. 111.

certain proportion of these cases of physiological disturbance trace more or less directly to the child's psychosexual development. A psychosomatic origin may also be found for some instances of disturbed physical growth. But we should not be too confident that all or even a majority of the physiological and physical anomalies which occur in adolescence have a primarily psychological source. The child's reaction to these apparent anomalies, the extent to which he tolerates them or is deeply worried by them, is a psychological matter, but their source and incidence seem quite as likely to depend upon intrinsic factors in the biological growth pattern as upon factors in the family situation or in the child's personality structure.

It is difficult to discuss the physical aspects of adolescence without reference to the factor of timing, and to differences in the age at which the puberal growth cycle begins. Let us consider first the facts as to the timing of puberty, and then the bearing of these facts upon adolescent problems. We shall see that it is of the first importance to know not merely what bodily changes are brought about by puberal growth, but also when these changes are induced.

In the case of girls, the most commonly used landmark for recording individual differences in puberal maturing is the menarche or the time of first menstruation. This occurs, of course, relatively late in the puberal growth cycle: a little more than a year after the adolescent growth spurt has reached its peak, and a little more than three years after the beginning of the growth spurt.[9]

In our California sample the menarche coincides, on the average, with the beginning of the teen age, falling at thirteen years and one month. In some Eastern studies a somewhat later age has been indicated, nearer thirteen and a half or even fourteen. The question has been asked whether this difference is due to the stimulation of being near Hollywood, or whether it is an example of earlier maturing in a milder climate. The latter may be a fac-

---

[9] Frank K. Shuttleworth, *Sexual Maturation and the Physical Growth of Girls, Age Six to Nineteen* (Washington, D.C.: Society for Research in Child Development, 1937).

tor, but we should point out the error in the popular idea that adolescence comes earliest in the Tropics. Adolescence is probably earliest in the Temperate Zone, and arrives somewhat later as we go north into the colder regions or south into tropical countries. For example, in a recent study in South America,[10] the average age of menarche directly under the equator, both in the mountains and in coastal areas, and for different ethnic groups, was found to be retarded almost a full year as compared with our California records.

We cannot be sure, however, that this is related to climate in any direct way rather than to general socio-economic conditions and conditions of health. Unfavorable living standards apparently tend to retard the beginning of adolescence; recent observers of child development in war-stricken areas of Europe have been impressed by this fact. A related finding may be the tendency for American children in the same social groups to mature earlier in this generation than was true fifty or a hundred years ago.[11] This is probably an illustration of the complex, biosocial nature of adolescence; for while earlier maturing may be attributable to gains in health and nutrition, these, in turn, rest upon social trends.

There is an implication here which may be worth noting. One effect of civilized living has been to extend the term of social adolescence, by delaying the time at which young people can begin to earn their own living. As society becomes more complex, educational demands increase, and more years must be devoted to preparation for adult life. One effect of this has been, of course, to delay the age of marriage and to lengthen the period of sexual postponements or compromises. But social adolescence is also being lengthened at the other end, by pushing the time of maturing down to an earlier age. It is probably safe to say that the period of social adolescence is now from two to three times as long as was the case in America several generations ago. Thus the improved conditions for healthy physical growth, which our so-

---

[10] Ulises D. Arrieta, "Menstrual Biology of the Peruvian Woman," *La Cronica Medica*, XLIX, No. 332 (October, 1932), 277–87.
[11] Clarence A. Mills, *Medical Climatology* (Baltimore: Thomas, 1939).

ciety has gradually achieved, tend to make more difficult some of the adolescent problems of mental hygiene, because of the much greater length of time during which these problems must be faced.

Our chief purpose, however, is not to discuss the average age of maturing of various groups, but the great diversity within any group. In any normal sampling of schoolgirls we may expect to find some who reach the menarche at eleven years of age or even a little earlier; and some who are delayed until sixteen or even a little later. In terms of physical growth changes, some girls in a normal sample show the beginning of rapid puberal growth as early as nine years of age and others not until after twelve or thirteen. These extreme differences are not without important after effects. The early-maturing girl who reaches her peak of growth at eleven or even earlier also reaches an early limit of growth. By thirteen she has attained nearly her adult stature, and this adult stature is short.[12] The adolescent growth period is more or less abruptly brought to an end, epiphyses at the growing ends of the bones are closed, and no further increase in height is possible. If you plot the growth curves of early- and of late-maturing girls, you will find that the former are taller in childhood, even at six or seven years of age; they gain in relative height until the age of twelve, when they may be as much as four inches taller than the late-maturing, but by fifteen they are definitely in a shorter-than-average classification.

At the University of California we conducted a series of studies to determine the relationship of these early changes to problems of adjustment. In general, it appears that the very early-maturing girl, at least in an urban culture, is in many respects in a disadvantageous position. In one of our studies, not yet published, we selected two groups of early- and late-maturing girls, on the basis of skeletal maturity as read from X rays. These were not clinical deviates nor cases of endocrine pathology, but merely the physically most precocious 20 percent and the physically most re-

[12] Nancy Bayley, "Size and Body Build of Adolescents in Relation to Rate of Skeletal Maturing," *Child Development*, XIV, No. 2 (June, 1943), 47–90.

Shuttleworth, *The Physical and Mental Growth of Girls and Boys Age Six to Nineteen in Relation to Age at Maximal Growth*.

tarded 20 percent in a normal sample of girls from a public school. The two groups were similar in intelligence, in socio-economic status, in racial background, and in their childhood health records. When we compared them, however, with regard to various social traits, as noted by careful observers in a long series of records, we found that the early-maturing were below the average in prestige, sociability, and leadership; below the average in popularity; below the average in cheerfulness, poise, and expressiveness. In the opinion of their classmates, as judged from a reputation test, they were considered to be rather submissive, withdrawn, and lacking in assurance.

These deficiencies in social attitudes and behavior may indeed be interpretable in terms of deeper layers of personality, but before seeking a more recondite explanation we may point out certain obvious and external ways in which the early-maturing girl is handicapped. The first thing to note is that she finds that she has become physically very conspicuous, at a time when conspicuousness is not valued. She finds herself embarrassingly tall and heavy; she is embarrassed by a greater breast development than seems to her to be normal; she is handicapped when she attempts to participate in the active playground games which are still within the interests of her classmates—for in the case of girls, sexual maturing, although it brings greater strength, often leads to a decreased skill in physical activities involving running and jumping.

The early-maturing girl quite naturally has interests in boys and in social usages and activities more mature than those of her chronological age group. But the males of her own age are unreceptive, for while she is physiologically a year or two out of step with the girls in her class, she is three or four years out of step with the boys—a vast and terrifying degree of developmental distance.

Sometimes the early-maturing girl manages to escape into an older age group, and to associate with other adolescents in her neighborhood who are nearer her own physiological level. In doing this, however, she may encounter other problems that are even more serious. Some of these may be involved in the attitudes of her parents, who are scarcely prepared for this sudden jump into young womanhood. They may feel that she is not yet old enough to go to parties or to have "dates"; they may demand that she continue to dress and act like other eleven- or twelve-year-olds. In this they may have some slight justification; for, unfortunately, a physical growth spurt does not carry with it any corresponding spurt in mental growth, and the physiologically mature youngster may not have the judgment nor mental level which go with longer living. So she is caught in this dilemma: if she remains in her own age group she is frustrated and ill at ease; if she moves into an older group she may fall under parental restrictions and, in any event, may lack the social maturity necessary to make a good adjustment among others of greater experience. To a considerable extent these difficulties are due to the age-grade system of our public schools, which make a physiologically deviate child conspicuous among her classmates. This would be less likely to occur in a small modern school which can make flexible provisions for individuals or, indeed, in the old-time district school, in which the grades are mixed in a single room. A completely heterogeneous grouping, as in the latter instance, may have disadvantages from a teaching standpoint, but for both early- and late-maturing children it may carry great advantages from a social standpoint.

In the case of girls, however, the late-maturing appear to need no special aids or compensations, unless their growth lag is so great as to imply a pathological condition. In the study mentioned above, the girls who were late-maturing were not only superior to the early-maturing but also superior to the average in a great number of the characteristics included in our social observation schedules. They were significantly higher than the early-maturing in traits related to personal appearance and attractiveness, in expressiveness and activity, in buoyance, poise, and cheerfulness, and also in sociability, leadership, and prestige. We are here, of course, speaking of each group taken as a whole; individual cases can be found which do not by any means conform to these generalizations.

Several points may be noted in explaining the apparently

better status of so many of the late-maturing girls. The first is a physical advantage. Because of lateness in sexual maturing and in the closing of the epiphyses at the growing points of the bones, she has a long time in which to grow. Her growth is less sudden, less abrupt, than in the early-maturing, seldom reaches as great a velocity at the peak of growth, and involves fewer hazards of physiological imbalance and physical disproportion. The longer period of growth affects particularly the legs, and the late-maturing girl is therefore long-legged, and tends to conform closely to our American standards of beauty of figure, which in the present code of commercial advertising must always be long-legged and usually a bit hypofeminine.

Moreover, in this slower process of adolescence, the parents and the girl herself have a longer time in which to get used to the new interests, new impulses, and new requirements as to behavior. One further point is probably rather important. The late-maturing girl is more nearly in step with the boys in her age group than is the case with the early- or average-maturing girl. The two-year lag in the average maturity patterns of boys as compared with girls is reduced or eliminated among those girls who mature late, and their interests in mixed social activities, when they emerge, are more immediately satisfied.

If now we consider what adolescence may mean to the early- or the late-maturing boy, we find results quite the reverse of those reported for girls. The early-maturing boy enters adolescence at a time when girls in his age group are appreciative of male acquaintances who no longer insist upon being children. He also acquires traits of strength and athletic ability which give him prestige with his own sex. He is likely to be nearer the Apollonian build than the boys who mature later. He wins friends and influences people through the mere fact of physiological precocity, and through the physical dominance which follows.[13]

This is, of course, not without its hazards. The hazard lies partly in discrepancies in different aspects of growth, and discrepancies between what a boy is prepared to do and what his parents

[13] Harold E. Jones, *Motor Performance and Growth* (Berkeley: University of California Press, 1949).

and other adults expect and demand of him. The boy who at thirteen is as tall as an adult may be assigned tasks beyond his years. His teacher chooses him for positions of responsibility. The athletic coach grooms him for the first team. His parents expect him to carry a larger share of the family burdens. A thirteen-year-old may not be ready for all this. Muscular development tends to lag somewhat behind skeletal development, and although he is strong, the early-maturing boy is not so strong as he looks. These new demands fall upon him at a time when he is already carrying a heavy load of adjustment to a changed physical structure, a new body image, and new interests and impulses. Nevertheless, in spite of these handicaps, and his very rapid rate of physical change, the early-maturing boy may readily find more advantages than disadvantages in his position. Moreover, unlike the physically precocious girl, his growth is not arrested at an early age; he reaches an average height as an adult, and somewhat better than average strength and general physical ability.

On the other hand, the boy who matures late, like the girl who matures early, is out of step with all the others in his age group. At fifteen or even sixteen he may still be a little boy, ignored by other boys and girls alike, and unable to compete effectively in playground games. In my book *Development in Adolescence*,[14] I have presented an example of such a case, a boy who developed many subjective inferiorities in connection with his retarded maturing, and whose compensation took the form of an ineffective social striving. Many of our late-maturing boys adjust by withdrawing from competition, becoming submissive and self-effacing. Others may take a more positive line of action; these are the active small boys, noisy, aggressive, and attention-getting. When at long last the late-maturing boy attains his growth spurt he is likely to reach normal height, but he may be slow to recover from the psychological scars of the period when he was a deviate. Such boys can be helped by giving them a prediction of their adult height and of the time when they may expect to enter the puberal phase of rapid growth. On the basis of Bayley's work, we

[14] Harold E. Jones, *Development in Adolescence: Approaches to the Study of the Individual* (New York: Appleton-Century, 1943).

can now make this prediction, from skeletal X rays, with a fair degree of accuracy.[15] The boy's pressing but often unasked question, "Am I normal?" can usually be answered in the affirmative. He can be more patient in waiting for nature to take its course, if he understands that his difficulty is merely one of timing and not of basic deficiency.

We have mentioned the sex difference in puberal maturing, which inducts girls into adolescence a year or two earlier, on the average, than boys. Another sex difference has been pointed out from one of our other studies by Dr. Caroline Tryon. Achieving manhood or womanhood in our society,

is a long, complex, and often confusing learning task. . . . For the most part boys and girls work at these tasks in a stumbling, groping fashion, blindly reaching for the next step without much or any adult assistance. Many lose their way. It seems probable that our adult failure to give assistance derives as much from ignorance about this developmental process as it does from the extensive taboos on sex which characterize our culture.[16]

One of the aspects of this developmental process is that, at least in an urban American culture, girls appear to have a greater problem than boys in adjusting to changing social requirements. In the adolescent culture itself girls encounter many changes in the conception as to what constitutes desirable behavior, changes and even reversals in the value system and in the relative ranking of traits which are important for popularity and prestige. Perhaps the principal single change which we have found in our California group is that at the beginning of adolescence the group standards for conduct among girls emphasize a quiet, demure, rather lady-like demeanor. By the age of fifteen this has altered, and we find that the girls who are now most popular in their set are active, talkative, and marked by a kind of "aggressive good fellowship." These traits, which may in part be adaptations to the hesitant and immature social approaches of boys, must

---

[15] Nancy Bayley, "Tables for Predicting Adult Heights from Skeletal Age and Present Heights," *Journal of Pediatrics*, XXVIII, No. 1 (January, 1946), 49–64.
[16] Caroline M. Tryon, "The Adolescent Peer Culture," in *Forty-third Yearbook of the National Society for the Study of Education* (Chicago: Chicago University, Department of Education, 1944), Part I, "Adolescence," p. 234.

again undergo considerable change in the later years of adolescence, if a girl is to maintain her status in the group. Dr. Tryon points out that boys, by comparison, seem to have a somewhat more consistent set of criteria to meet in developing their sex roles during this growth period.

While there are many other aspects of social adjustment which should be discussed in considering adolescence in our culture, I shall limit myself to one additional topic. I should like to discuss one of our investigations of social adjustment in a wider reference, the adjustment not merely to one's own group, but to members of other groups. We are all keenly aware that this is one of the important problems facing us, in developing and maintaining the conditions for democratic living in our society.

In a field research now under way, we have attempted to make a comparison between children and youth in the adolescent period who are markedly prejudiced toward members of various alien or minority groups, and adolescents who fall at the other extreme of tolerance, accepting and respecting the values and ways of life of others even when these characteristics are quite different from their own. In this study we have obtained rather extensive case records for children representing the most prejudiced 25 percent and the least prejudiced 25 percent, in a total group of about fifteen hundred school children.

The most prejudiced are presumably those who, in any group, provide the most vigorous drive and support for ethnocentric and, in that sense, antidemocratic, doctrines and activities. They are the ones who are least ready for any sort of world citizenship. Among their social attitudes, quoting from results which have been formulated by Dr. Frenkel-Brunswik,[17] we find a tendency to revere the strong and dominating and to despise those who are weak. This seems readily to extend to an exaltation of the ingroup and a rejection of any out-group, including those who are foreign or are presumed to be socially inferior. The prejudiced child does a great deal of projecting and blaming others, finding scapegoats. He often has a feeling of being victimized, of living

[17] E. Frenkel-Brunswik. "A Study of Prejudice in Children," *Human Relations*, I, No. 3 (1948), 295–306.

in a world in which there are many subtle and evil people, and also of being threatened with many physical dangers.

Along with this, the prejudiced boy inclines toward ideals of aggressive toughness. His conception of masculinity has strong components, not only of vigor, but also of harshness and violence. Girls, on the other hand, must keep within narrow limits of feminine passivity. Their place is at home, and evidences of tomboyishness or even independence should be frowned upon. The members of the opposite sex are, in effect, regarded by these boys as an out-group. It would seem that tolerance of the opposite sex, and an equalitarian relationship between the sexes, has an important bearing upon tolerance in general.

If we ask how these attitudes have developed, we can give as yet no fully satisfactory description of the process, but we have been somewhat impressed by the discovery that the prejudiced children have been reared in families in which there exists, on the average, a more rigid discipline than in families at the unprejudiced extreme; more rigid discipline and also, perhaps, a certain lack of affection. A child can stand strict discipline if he feels that his parents really love him, but if their love is conditional, if it is something that can be turned on or off according to whether he is "good" or "bad," he is likely to feel a more fundamental frustration than would be involved merely in discipline taken by itself. We would state the matter thus: Frustration is obviously impossible to avoid. Every child as he grows older encounters new and more complex frustrations which he must learn to assimilate if he is to become socialized. But the way in which frustration is imposed by the parent may have important consequences for the child's personality.

It seems a reasonable hypothesis that one form of adjustment to too rigid and too unloving a discipline is to accept this discipline, to conform, and outwardly to identify with the strict ideals of the parents, but at the same time to develop a repressed resentment. The child cannot express his resentment toward his own family nor toward members of the dominant in-group. Instead, he expresses it, often in quite intensified form, toward out-groups, toward those who are foreign or who seem to him to be socially or biologically inferior. These repressed hostile tendencies may be attached unrealistically, not merely to other people, but also to natural phenomena—our prejudiced children are not only more afraid of human enemies in many subtle and dangerous forms, but they are also more afraid of disease germs, of violent storms, and, in California, of earthquakes.

Another point that has been noted about many of the families of our prejudiced children is that they seem to be very status-concerned, concerned about their position in society, in terms of the external appearances of status. They seem to communicate to their children a set of somewhat rigid, externalized, and superficial values which reflect their own preoccupations. As a result, the children tend to appraise others in terms of quite arbitrary criteria of power or weakness, conformity or difference, being clean or not being clean, knowing the right people or not knowing the right people. Perhaps connected with these processes is a tendency for the prejudiced child to be more rigid in many of his mental processes, not merely in his attitude toward minority groups, but in his attitudes toward acquaintances with whom he rarely has a close personal relationship, toward social events, political ideas, and even in the way he does his abstract thinking.

We have touched on only a few aspects of adolescence in our society. The motive in this selection has not been to cover the whole range of topics or, necessarily, the most important ones, but to discuss a few of the problem areas with which we must deal. Some of these are primarily social, others primarily biological in origin, but they all become expressed in the adjustment of the adolescent as a biosocial organism. There was a time when we referred quite frequently to the Four Freedoms. For the adolescent there must be another freedom, the freedom to become adult. Modern society imposes many restrictions on this freedom, and throws many hazards and delays in the path of growing up. Our own task as adults is to lend the adolescent a helping hand as he struggles toward maturity, always remembering, however, that it is he who must do the growing, and in his own way.

The Adaptive Problems of the Adolescent Personality

NATHAN W. ACKERMAN, M.D.

THE PSYCHOLOGICAL DISTURBANCES OF THE TEEN AGE represent an age-old enigma. Some parts of this enigma are solved; others still await an answer. Despite the crucial importance of adolescent phenomena for the process of maturation, even now they are not yet fully understood. The ever changing forms and subtle instabilities of adolescent behavior are unique and lend a peculiarly elusive quality to the adolescent personality. Occasionally, the real meaning of these evanescent reactions escapes even the more astute observers. It is small wonder, then, that these problems have always stirred the interest and imagination of students of human nature. Among these, caseworkers and psychiatrists have a special stake; for them, a clear understanding of adolescence is of immense theoretical and practical importance.

The social conduct of adolescents can be most trying. It can impose the severest test on the surrounding environment, particularly the immediate environment of the family. To meet that test successfully, the environment must be both stable and healthy. It is common knowledge that parents too often fail to understand such behavior. They often react in exactly the wrong way. Sometimes, they fear the worst, as, for example, the beginning of a hardened criminal career, or even a psychosis, when actually the child is experiencing a temporary adolescent storm from which he will emerge intact, unscarred, and with reasonably good mental health. Or, parents come to the psychiatrist grudgingly, suspiciously, insisting that the child's difficulties are merely expressions of "normal adolescence," when actually the child has a serious personality defect.

To misunderstand the meaning of adolescent conduct may sometimes have serious consequences. A parent who vacillates, who alternately indulges and disciplines a disturbed adolescent, may do crucial harm to the process of maturation. We shall try to show why, particularly in the adolescent era, the danger from confusion and misinterpretation is so great.

The community, as well as the parent, carries a large responsibility for setting the stage for the adolescent's struggle with the tasks of adult living. Social agencies, in their organic closeness to community organization, have a fundamental concern with the issues of adolescent adaptation. This is concretely reflected in organized efforts to prevent delinquency, to provide educational, recreational, and vocational guidance, and, finally, systematic psychotherapy.

But there is one unique reason for the interest of caseworkers in adolescence, especially the younger workers. Close in age, and fresh from the struggle themselves, they engage in an intimate, though not always admitted, identification with the conflicts, fears, and aspirations of adolescents. Caseworkers, as a group, enjoy a special gift in the treatment of the emotional disturbances of adolescents. It has been for me a gratifying experience to see the astoundingly good therapeutic results often achieved by workers in treating adolescents.

For psychiatrists, obviously, the vicissitudes of adolescent behavior have fundamental significance. Out of the fiery crucible of adolescent change is precipitated, not only the permanent structure of the adult personality, but also the major forms of mental disease. Adolescence is a normal crisis in the growth process; it is also the deepest crisis in the growth process. The personality undergoes a basic shift in equilibrium, characterized by simultaneous tendencies toward disorganization and reorganization. Out of these transitional processes finally emerges the permanent configuration of personality. During this period, the culture exercises a profound shaping influence on personality; it selectively reinforces or weakens specific character tendencies. Intense conflict emerges at all levels of the emotional life. The earlier disturbances of personality are reactivated; latent weak-

Adaptive Problems of Adolescence

nesses are exposed. Dispositions toward specific psychiatric illnesses are reinforced; the major psychiatric disorders of adult life may be precipitated. An accurate understanding of the psychodynamics of adolescence is indispensable for correct insight into all categories of psychopathology.

The typical manifestations of adolescent change are familiar to all of us: the pervasive insecurity; the instability of mood and action; the egocentricity; the prominence of the sexual drives; the exhibitionism; the loyalty to the same sex and the fear and suspicion of the opposite sex; the confusion; the shifting concepts of self, the self-consciousness; the lack of ease with one's own body; the preoccupation with physique and health; the vulnerability of self-esteem; the exaggerated feelings of difference; the conflict concerning authority, social forces, religion, and philosophy; the rebelliousness; the craving for independence; the obstinacy; the hero worship and the suggestibility to outside influence; the fear of inadequacy and failure; the tendency to depression and social withdrawal; and, finally, the aspiration to be outstanding in some field of human achievement.

Underlying these rapid, radical shifts of behavior are the fundamental, biological processes of pubescence. Changes in glandular function produce changes in physique, in physiological balance; with these changes, the sex drives emerge.

The growth processes tend to be asymmetrical. The physical changes do not always take a sex-appropriate course. There is a spurt in physical growth, both in height and weight. In girls, there is the onset of menses, the change in contour of the body, the development of breasts and hips, changes in skin texture, and, frequently, acne. In boys, there is the growth of the genitals, the onset of ejaculation, change in voice, hair growth, and skin texture, and acne.

Throughout, the elements of physical change are accompanied by a shift in emotional, social, sexual, and intellectual behavior. Inequalities of development in these various spheres tend to intensify the usual instability. Not only are there tremendous variations from one individual to the next, but, perhaps even more important, every conceivable type of imbalance may occur within the one individual, a factor which sharply stimulates anxiety, self-consciousness, feelings of difference and inferiority.

Overt sexual desire emerges in both sexes. Masturbation is more easily stimulated in boys than in girls. Girls develop earlier their secondary sexual characteristics, but are slower in their actual sexual awakening. For boys, sex offers its own intrinsic pleasures; for girls, in this society, sex has traditionally represented a means to an end, rather than an end in itself; that is, the sexual behavior of girls is closely linked to strivings for security and prestige. But this, too, is changing; for girls it is also becoming sex for the sake of sex.

We have characterized adolescence as a critical stage of development in which the anatomic unity of personality is temporarily dismembered and reformed. All sorts of transitional adaptation between childhood and adulthood appear. Adolescence, therefore, is an in-between phenomenon reflecting features both of the child and adult. But, adolescence has positive features of its own. Phenomenonologically, it is certainly not a clear-cut entity; yet it is characterized by one dramatically positive feature, sexual maturation. Adolescence can be defined as the series of changes in personality adaptation impelled by sexual differentiation and maturation, which, in turn, are conditioned by the surrounding cultural pattern. The complex of adolescent behavior is thus the product, on the one hand, of the impact of growth changes, with particular emphasis on the sexual changes of pubescence and, on the other hand, of the pressure of cultural forces. The pressures from within and without the personality squeeze the structure of the self between them. This two-way assault inexorably forces a profound change in the equilibrium of personality, and accounts for the simultaneous dissolution and resolution of the adolescent's self. The emergence of an unbalanced mixture of childhood and adult traits is, therefore, to be expected. The adolescent does not mature in a consistent forward movement; instead, anxiety (which is ever present) induces an irregular movement, alternately forward and backward. The adolescent loses the protection of childhood, but does not yet have the strength and privileges of the adult. The realities of adult living

Adaptive Problems of Adolescence

represent still an unknown and undefined menace. Fear of being a child pushes the adolescent forward. Fear of being an adult pushes him backward. Dangers loom large either in moving toward maturity or in regressing to childhood forms of adaptation.

The closeness of the adolescent to his group life is a significant molding force during this transitional adaptation. Often, the interchange between the adolescent and his group is so fluid and rich that the respective identities of the adolescent and his group can hardly be separated. The distinction, therefore, between what is properly inside and outside the adolescent self cannot always be clear. Within the family circle, the adolescent rebels. Outside the family, the need of the adolescent to conform to dominant group standards is often extreme. The adolescent is expected, during this period of transition, to "find himself." There is a great danger, however, of losing himself, through an exaggerated, submissive need for conformity. The adolescent may either dissolve himself into the activities of the surrounding group, or defensively isolate himself. This may signify either a positive group identification, or a negative effort toward self-preservation through isolation. Thus, in the end, the adolescent may solidify his individuality, or submerge it behind defensive conformity.

Culture, in all times, has played a large role in dictating the adolescent's place in the social scheme, and in shaping adolescent personality. Culture, for the adolescent, comprises a far wider group of cultural influences than those which surround the child. The adolescent moves out and makes contact with an expanding variety of groups bound by common religious, recreational, intellectual, and economic interests. In all societies, adolescents achieve new privileges, but they must assume new responsibilities. They are called upon to demonstrate their worth socially, sexually, economically. They are expected to pursue and control their sexual drives according to modes predetermined by the given culture. They must evolve into approved versions of men and women. Beyond this point, generalizations become difficult. Each individual society imposes a distinct set of standards. The discrepancies between one society and another are often striking. Moreover, within any single large culture, such as our own, there are infinite numbers of subcultures ("island cultures," so called) which, in turn, among themselves reflect sharp differences in standards. In accordance with these differential characteristics, each society ushers in adolescence with a unique set of social customs. Initiation ceremonies and rituals, richly symbolic in content, fix the time and conditions of transition to adulthood. It is a familiar historical fact that earlier societies often inflicted painful physical ordeals on adolescents; such was the price of admission to adult society. The ability to endure successfully these physical ordeals signified proof of readiness for the assumption of adult tasks.

The effects of culture on personality have varied through the ages. In this respect, past and present social systems are sharply contrasted. Earlier societies were often less complex in pattern, but more rigid. Cultural influences tended to be more definite, more static, more consistent. The established patterns of social and sexual conduct were sharply delineated. The dominant taboos were unmistakable. The price of achieving adulthood was impressed on adolescents in a manner not to be denied. The adolescent's task of assimilating cultural standards was then presumably easier. The role of present-day culture is more difficult to assay. The standards of modern society are extremely unstable and contradictory. This is one inevitable expression of the vast social crisis which is the outstanding feature of our time in history. Revolutionary forces are irresistibly chipping away at established patterns of social organization. A radical metamorphosis of social aims and values is the inevitable concomitant of this crucial change in our dominant social institutions. As a result, standards are inconsistent, confused, at times frankly chaotic, or, occasionally, simply nonexistent. In such times, safe standards are difficult to find.

This process filters down even to the smallest subcultures, and has a profound effect on the stability of family life. The unity of the family, parental attitudes, child rearing, the vicissitudes of personality maturation, the formation of conscience, are all

Adaptive Problems of Adolescence

deeply affected. Guilt reactions, in this culture, tend to show a peculiarly inconsistent and fickle character. Against this background, it is easy to understand the unique vulnerability of adolescent emotional life to the chaos which features our social order.

The moral code with which children are indoctrinated is not the same as that which dominates the scene in adult society. Children who are taught to share, to coöperate, to be truly considerate of the rights of other persons, are ill prepared for the code of ruthless competitive aggression which prevails in the adult world.

Present-day society places an inordinately high premium on success—success in conventional prestige tones, success at any price. The unrestrained, crude use of aggression proves often to be a sheer necessity for the achievement of conventional success. The aggressiveness must be efficient in its ruthless stamping out of rivals. The pattern of conscience structured in childhood, however, reacts to such aggression with intense anxiety, fear of retaliation, fear of being hated and ostracized. It can hardly be a surprise, then, that so many so-called "successful" adults feel isolated and have little sense of really belonging anywhere. One conspicuous characteristic of modern society is its impoverished group life; members of our society have little opportunity for experiencing a positive sense of security in their group affiliations. This has an obvious and immediate relevance to the adolescent's struggle for acceptance, and for a solid sense of his own identity.

One other feature of our culture compounds the difficulties of adolescent adaptation, that is, the highly developed technology and the trend toward specialization. The necessity for long apprenticeship, in preparation for the special tasks of adult life, imposes on the adolescent a status of prolonged dependence. It tends to intensify his struggle with feelings of inadequacy; this prolongation of training, together with the forced economic dependence, hampers his sexual maturation.

Thus, in contrast with earlier forms of society, the pattern of interaction between the adolescent and his surrounding culture is today not so clearly defined. The adolescent has little security with surrounding groups. The interrelationship is vague and menacing in its uncertainty. The opportunities are ill defined, the dangers great. There are not the familiar guideposts that adolescents of older generations got from their parents. The adolescent today never knows exactly what to expect, or where he stands.

The adolescent, seeking an individuality separate and distinct from that of his parents, ventures out into wider spheres. Inevitably disillusioned in the standards of his parents, he searches for new and more satisfying standards. From among these diverse extrafamilial groups, he may make a choice. He does so in accordance with the vicissitudes of his changing concept of self and the outer world. To replace the shattered ideal of his parents, he seeks a new ideal. The unusual features of modern society render the adolescent's problem of choice more difficult and complex. Society offers little by way of positive guidance. The group life of adolescents today is woefully lacking in real substance. Neighborhood centers for youth are tragically deficient in inspired leadership appropriate to adolescent need. The emotional atmosphere of such centers only too often is conspicuously colorless and void of appeal. By contrast, the human atmosphere of the bowling alley or the neighborhood poolroom, balefully regarded as breeding places for adolescent crime, sometimes reflect more basic understanding of the emotional strivings of adolescents than do the respected neighborhood centers. Such places could well be exploited as neighborhood clubs with community interests and a social code suited to adolescent needs. The natural formation of adolescent groups into so-called "cellar clubs," usefully exploited by well-trained leaders, might easily be a significant cultural force for good. There is great advantage in preserving spontaneous groupings of adolescents wherever one finds them. The possibilities for constructive guidance of adolescents, utilizing these natural groups, have hardly been touched.

This poverty of opportunity for gratifying self-expression in group life is responsible for another significant trend in adolescent behavior, namely, the adolescent striving to create his own culture, to mold social realities to his own liking. Some features of current society tend strongly to activate this tendency. Adoles-

Adaptive Problems of Adolescence

cents try hard to create within their own group a small world of their own, with unique standards and values, carefully suited to their needs. They make a place for themselves if the world outside fails them. To whatever extent they do not feel accepted, they will withdraw and create their own separate community within the larger community. This trend is akin to the attitude of eccentrics, utopians, artists, and writers who, uncomfortable under the pressure of ordinary social realities, which they feel are hostile and unsympathetic, withdraw and create their own community. They endeavor to create a new social group, more closely fitting their special needs. Here is the effort to lock off a smaller world within a larger one—to fence off an "island culture." Whether fortunate or otherwise, this is never really successful. At best, such efforts are only partly or temporarily successful. In the end, interpenetration between the "island culture" and the parent culture inevitably occurs, and the challenge of "one world" demands an answer. This defensive group behavior of adolescents must be regarded as a reflection of the failure of the parent culture to provide an adequate place for the expression of adolescent personality.

The influence of these wider group affiliations molds the social and sexual conduct of adolescence. But this is a two-way process: the culture molds the adolescent, but the adolescent also molds the culture. These and other phases of the interaction of the adolescent with his surrounding culture, which I cannot go into here, condition his drive for emancipation from authority, heterosexual success, and achievement in the intellectual, social, and economic spheres. Even in the most favored of circumstances, this struggle is characterized by strain, conflict, confusion, and insecurity. From it finally emerges the more stable adult pattern of interpersonal relations.

Now, let us turn our attention exclusively to the inner factors, the intrapsychic vicissitudes of adolescence. It is a period of diffuse conflict, having pervasive effects on all levels of personality functioning. The phenomena of adolescence embrace all aspects of the personality. The disorders of this period are of the total personality; they do not represent pathology in the sexual area alone. Some adolescents recoil from meeting the vital issues; others take a headlong plunge into them. It should be remembered, however, that such a plunge may signify merely a further effort in disguise to avoid contact with the real problems.

What of the oft-repeated statement that adolescence is par excellence the stage of reactivation of oedipal conflict? This is the truth, but not the whole truth. While the oedipal issues and identity conflicts may occupy the center of the stage, the fact is that all the significant conflict areas are reactivated. It cannot be otherwise. The fluidity of the concepts of self, the changing aims and aspirations, the instability of repression, the effort to rebuild a conscience suited to maturity, the imperious quality of the sex drives, bring into sharp focus every conflict, past and present, which has failed to achieve solution. All this adds up to one central feature, the understanding of which is indispensable for correct interpretation of any and all manifestations of adolescence, namely, the instability and vulnerability of the adolescent personality. At no period in life do human beings feel as exposed and defenseless as in adolescence. The protective coloring of the personality is stripped off, and the deeper emotional currents are laid bare. Thus is made evident the diffuse, pervasive anxiety, the sense of exposure, the embarrassment and self-consciousness. This is the matrix on which is nourished the adolescent's belligerent defense of his privacy.

Illustration: A boy of fifteen; the only son of a scientist. He has a soft, delicate, somewhat feminine face. He is confused about sexual matters, has feelings of inferiority about his physique, and some submerged anxiety about homosexuality. His manner is detached. He treats people with an air of aloofness and constraint. His parents have been separated since he was seven years of age. His mother made adamant demands that he make his home with her. He bitterly rejected these demands, and insisted on living with his father, but he allowed neither parent to intrude into any aspect of his personal life. He was Sphinxlike in his obstinate determination to shut out both parents. He exercised, literally, a twenty-four hour vigilance over his privacy, to such an extent that both parents knew almost nothing of his personal feelings, interests, and activities. At home with his father, his facial expression was a mask; he was reticent, maintained a strict

Adaptive Problems of Adolescence

isolation. When his father made an effort to show interest in his private affairs, he reacted belligerently and insolently. He visited his mother occasionally, when he could not avoid it, and maintained the same silent guard with her. Outside his family, his manner was distinctly less suspicious, more agreeable and friendly.

Defenses against anxiety in adolescence reflect this generalized instability and vulnerability. They operate inefficiently; they appear in dramatic and extreme form; they are readily transparent; there are rapid shifts from one pattern of defense to another.

We turn now to a consideration of the multiple levels of conflict. There are conflicts revolving around the issue of self-assertion and self-esteem. These are reflected in a clash between real and ideal images of the self, and also as discrepancies between aspiration and actual achievement. There are conflicts between old and new patterns of conscience; also conflicts surrounding the expression of basic emotional and sexual needs, and the corresponding aggression.

Of first importance is the adolescent's effort to achieve a feeling of adequacy. Every single aspect of the adolescent's effort to adapt to reality is influenced by his sense of worth and confidence, or the lack of it. The actual experience of success, and the achievement of a feeling of strength and mastery in coping with the issues of life, is essential for good emotional balance. Lack of confidence, anxiety about adequacy, and fear of failure release a host of secondary defensive attitudes, among which we must group timidity, submissiveness, gullibility, or, at the other extreme, excessive rebellion, belligerence, the urge to intimidate others, and a variety of compensatory tendencies. Adolescents characteristically have a difficult time organizing their aggressive impulses. It is not easy for them to achieve stable integration. They do not know quite how to handle their aggressions, when to be assertive, or when to be yielding.

Illustration: A sixteen-year-old boy, with superior native endowment, who shows a striking discrepancy between his potential abilities and actual achievement. His achievement was practically nil. He frankly confessed that he had no ambition except to be a bum. His father was an outstanding success professionally, but the patient did not expect to accomplish anything in life. He insisted that he was interested only in the fun he could have now. He claimed this choice to be his own prerogative; so long as he stayed by himself and hurt no one else, why could he not simply be a bum if he so chose?

This boy persistently rejected responsibilities, dissipated his energies, refused any and all exertions, and fortified a pattern of passive resistance to authority. At school, he was a chronic failure academically and socially. He was strongly disliked by his peers because of his supercilious, patronizing, sarcastic attitude. He seized any opportunity to ridicule his schoolmates.

This was his conscious behavior. He attempted in every way to fortify this perverseness. Actually, he was unable to get real pleasure from any normal activity. Beneath his overt defensive attitudes, he was extremely tense, depressed, despairing, had death fears and a profound sense of defeat and inferiority. His self-esteem had been deeply hurt years back by a recognition that his successful, ambitious, vain father did not prize him for himself, but wished merely to pad his own vanity by exhibiting the boy's intellectual superiority. He insisted that the boy be twice as smart as any other boy. At the same time, the father never really got close to him emotionally. He was too detached and more absorbed in his professional activity than in his children. This is the background in which the boy built up his pattern of spite and negativism.

These emotional vicissitudes are easily recognizable as a phase of the adolescent's identity conflict, his struggle to resolve his identification with his parents and, from this, to build an individual identity uniquely his own. The manner in which the adolescent solves the oedipal struggle and builds his own identity influences basic aspects of his behavior; his aggressive pattern, his sexual tendencies, his attitude toward his own nature, and the nature of the world around him. The uncertainty and confusion, which characterize transitionally the adolescent's sense of his own self, radiate outward to affect all of the adolescent's attitudes toward life. It is a groping, questioning stage. The adolescent asks: "What is life? Who am I? What am I here for? Do I have a place in this world? Where do I fit? What is my importance in the larger scheme of things? To what groups shall I attach myself? Who are my real friends? Who are my enemies? Where must I fight? With whom? Against whom? For what kind of life goals?" And, finally: "Is life really worth the struggle?"

Adaptive Problems of Adolescence

This kind of feverish, anxious searching for identity and orientation is paralleled by the expanding adolescent interest in social and economic conflicts, in religion and philosophy. A good deal of vague, intellectual groping often characterizes this quest for orientation. Intellectual defenses are commonly exploited in the effort to lessen underlying anxiety. All these struggles deeply affect the adolescent's choice of group affiliations.

From a purely objective standpoint, religious and economic beliefs represent distinct entities. From the point of view of the adolescent's psychic life, however, the symbolic roles of these distinct fields of interest have much in common. The adolescent, in a time of rejection of parental images and temporary dissolution of self, seeks to identify with something larger than himself. His urge is to ally himself with a cause far greater than his own. Economic and religious groups offer such an opportunity. The allegiance to a group characterized by a special economic philosophy, especially one advocating social reform, or even revolution, serves to conceal the disappointment in parents, and to reinforce the unstable repression of hostility to parental authority. It also buttresses the unstable repression of adolescent sexual drives. The excessive religiosity of adolescents, or, on the other hand, their radical turn from it to atheism, is alleged often to be motivated by the need to strengthen the repression of unconscious, passive, dependent, homosexual strivings. To illustrate concretely, a strong parallel suggests itself between the fervor of submission to a new religion and the emotion of passive submission to homosexual seduction. Conversion to a new religion, or a new social ideal, may conceal an unconscious fear of homosexual leanings. Is this, however, the only significance of the adolescent's preoccupation with religion or with social philosophy? Can we not, in addition, view this in the positive sense as a stage in the expansion of the self, a legitimate quest for union with the larger world outside? Could this, perhaps, be profitably used for constructive social purposes?

Illustration: A nineteen-year-old boy was referred to the clinic after he had ignominiously flunked out of the first year of college. When asked why he wanted to go to college, he gave an incredibly vague reply: "I suppose, to do good for others." Further questioning failed to elicit any more concrete explanation of his motivation or life goal. Discussion of other aspects of his life revealed that this vagueness characterized all his actions and relationships. If nothing better showed up, he thought he would finally enter his father's business. His guiding principle was to do things "the easiest way." He disliked exertion.

This young man was detached, passive, wore a peculiar grin. His mother was a social worker of the old vintage; his father, a businessman. They were high up in the economic scale. They were assimilated Jews; all aspects of their social living reflected a strong, conformist trend. But the family life, emotionally, was drab, colorless, lacking in real substance. The mother, nominally a Jew, attended a Protestant church and encouraged the boy to do likewise. At thirteen, at his own request, he was converted to Christianity. From his earliest days he had felt the compulsion to conform in order to insure social acceptance. In fact, he leaned over backward to the extent of deliberately shunning Jewish circles for fear that Christian groups would exclude him. Acceptance by a Christian group of boys provided a sublimated gratification for his need for male companionship, but enabled him, at the same time, to reject his Jewish father.

He had a long, hooked nose which he disliked. He linked the appearance of his nose with Jewishness. Three times between the ages of eleven and fifteen he broke it in apparent accidents. He planned to have plastic surgery done at the age of nineteen, but seemingly he could not wait until then to change the shape of his nose. This boy's sense of masculine adequacy was damaged; he had some unconscious homosexual leaning. He was deeply confused in his concept of self, and equally confused as to what his parents represented. Beset with inner doubts about himself, and troubled with violent, repressed hostility against both parents, he resorted to "playing dumb." Though very intelligent, he wore a mask with people and acted as though he were quite dull and uncomprehending. This was his defense against extreme hostility to his parents. He concealed his real emotions behind a façade of dull compliance and inconspicuous politeness. Unconsciously, he equated exertion with hostility, and therefore assumed this defensive external guise of extreme passivity and lack of initiative.

Some of the most conspicuous adolescent conflict centers in real or fancied injury to self-esteem. Adolescents show extraordinary sensitiveness concerning their concept of self. They react with trigger-like responsiveness to what they think of themselves and what others think of them. Since their image of self is in a state of

Adaptive Problems of Adolescence

flux, they are especially vulnerable to other persons' judgments. The issue of being approved or disapproved by others assumes a critical importance. Earlier discussion has already hinted at their sensitiveness concerning feelings of difference, not only from others, but also from themselves, since the rapid transformation of personality gives them little opportunity to gain familiarity with one stage of self before it is replaced by a new one. All this is a necessary reflection of the fluidity of the self-structure. Not only is the self currently exposed to attacks on self-esteem, but past assaults on the image of self are dramatically laid bare.

Adolescents often disclose, with astounding vividness, memories of deep, early injuries to their narcissism. They painfully relive these childhood hurts. They dread renewed assaults on these old, but exposed, wounds. Not infrequently, they perceive them consciously as new, fresh wounds. Of importance, in this connection, are the adolescents' fears of bodily attack, physical pain, consciousness of defect, feelings of inferiority. Sometimes their basic conviction is one of having been irreversibly damaged. While, in some part, these attitudes often represent castration fear, their basic scope is actually far wider. At deeper levels, they signify a threat of destruction to the total integrity of self. In this context, fears of being dominated, engulfed, crushed, even killed, find their appropriate place. Masochistic motivation is frequently woven into the context of such anxieties.

On this background, the compensatory drives can be readily understood; the urge to be big, powerful, to be "top dog," completely to obliterate all possible rivals, and to rely for such purposes on fantasies of omnipotence. Of special significance is the highly developed narcissism, the sensitive vanity, and the exhibitionistic drives of adolescents. The misplaced assertion of these compensatory drives often impels a neurotic adolescent to commit acts of delinquency.

Illustration: An eighteen-year-old boy, reared in an Orthodox Jewish home, intelligent, but on the brink of expulsion from college for poor academic work and chronic lateness. Most times, he appeared painfully bored, under constant strain, dirty, degraded in appearance. This boy was seriously confused; he was variably depressed and afflicted with obsessive rituals, associated with death anxiety. He felt imprisoned by these rituals and by the monotony of his daily obligations. He hated all routines; his resistance took the form of chronic lateness to all commitments in time: classes, appointments, retiring at a reasonable hour, etc. His whole struggle in life was to push backward against the clock. His primary tendency was to be submissive, but he fought against this with morose defiance, insolence, belligerence.

He found it impossible to go to sleep before one or two o'clock, and in the morning he could hardly be roused from sleep. Weekends, he slept until two or three o'clock in the afternoon. Sleeping, for him, was an experience of stupor—symbolic death. He had an obsessive anxiety about lying down, and resisted going to bed. For a time, he did not dare to kiss a girl. He was parasitically dependent on the companionship of boy friends, but covered this up by assuming with them a leader's role. In the context of this group activity, he engaged in certain delinquencies, such as truancy, stealing money, running away from home.

At one extreme, he treated himself like dirt; he felt profoundly degraded and worthless. At the other extreme, he assumed an arrogant, grandiose, contemptuous air, and was devastating in his criticism of others. He was deeply guilty about certain overt sexual interests in his mother and sister, yet was bullishly aggressive to both. He attempted to torment them. At the same time, he had thinly disguised homosexual anxieties.

This boy was the product of an overprotective, controlling, and seductive mother, and a more controlled, but obstinate, domineering father. He hated asking his father for anything. In his early years, he was an unusually good boy, submissive to his mother, fearful of his father. Later, he rebelled against his mother and found himself trapped in a violently ambivalent struggle for supremacy with his father.

He showed marked confusion in his sexual identity. His life goals were confused by his pattern of negativism, his deeply injured self-esteem, his self-degradation, and compensatory grandiosity.

Still another level of conflict has to do with the reformation of the conscience during adolescence. This aspect of the problem must be considered from several different angles: the transformation of childhood to adult conscience; the conflict between impulse and conscience during adolescence with special reference to sexual drives, aggression, and themes of self-punishment; and, finally, the tendency to "externalize" the functions of conscience

Adaptive Problems of Adolescence

during adolescence, with the resulting tendency to "act out." These phases are not really distinct, but are interrelated aspects of a single phenomenon.

The tendency to "externalize" the functions of conscience reflects two opposite and conflicting urges: the temptation to deny personal responsibility for impulsive actions; and the need to be restrained from such actions by external prohibitive force, emanating from the parent or a substitute authority figure. The adolescent seeks this external limitation, because of his temporary inner deficiency of impulse control. Adolescents who fear the impetuousness of their own primitive urges are often relieved by, and grateful for, such protective restraint.

Illustration: A fifteen-year-old girl, large for her years, inhibited, shy, socially withdrawn, unable to make friends. She had a beautiful face that clashed cruelly with her figure. In physique, she alternated in appearance between something like a cadaver and the fat woman of the circus. At one time she weighed 88 pounds and looked like a walking corpse. At another time, she weighed 220 pounds, and looked like a freak. Either she nibbled food constantly and insatiably, or she put herself rigidly on a starvation diet.

She feared sex, and strictly avoided boys. She was, at the same time, intensely anxious, even greedy, in her sex interests. In fantasy, she characterized certain foods as feminine, others as masculine. She alternated between devouring one or the other type of food. She was confused as to how much she wanted to be a girl and attractive to boys, or to be strong, independent, and aggressive like boys.

She was not secure in her dependence on either parent. She had cannibalistic fantasies of eating her father's genital; then, overwhelmed with guilt, she punished herself with a starvation diet. But her basic hostility against her mother distorted this relationship too. She repressed this hostility and intensified her dependence on her mother, in order to reinforce her restraint of her sexual cravings. In this manner, she made her mother serve as an external conscience. Her conception of herself was so confused that she did not dare let herself grow up; she avoided the issues of maturity and clung tenaciously to the status of child.

During adolescence the guilt reactions are peculiarly labile. At first, they are rather rigid, and are clearly based on the pattern of moral standards laid down in childhood, the behavior being strongly controlled by the established trends of parental approval and disapproval. The temptation to transgress this code is accompanied by fear of punishment and loss of love of the parents. As the adolescent detaches himself from his parents, he shifts his dependence to persons and groups outside the family—occasionally, to other adults, but more conspicuously to peers and older adolescents who symbolize the "big brother or sister." Simultaneously, there takes place a corresponding shift in ideals and standards. New patterns of aspiration emerge, based on these new affiliations. Persons other than parents are now made to personify ideals and conscience. The adolescent tends to externalize his conflict and control his behavior in accordance with his need of acceptance by particular persons and groups outside the family. For a time, the standards laid down by peers and "big brothers" may completely dominate the adolescent's life, and thus bring about a severe clash with the parents' ideas about life. This subjective struggle over standards is often bitter because of the adolescent's fear of losing control over his sexual and aggressive urges. The temptation to release these drives is intense, but the adolescent, dreading the loss of control, clings tenaciously to his childhood conscience and the parent from whom it was derived. These symbols represent for him a safe haven. This is the expression of adolescent conservatism and caution. But adolescents vacillate; they swing from one extreme to the other; they tend either to be overcautious and rigid, or positively rash.

In this period of unstable transformation, there are lightning shifts of behavior characterized alternately by restraint and self-indulgence. Strivings which represent elements of unconscious conflict are released impulsively. Inevitably, such "acting out" is followed by a resurgence of guilt and anxiety, and this, in turn, impels the reimposition, temporarily at least, of childhood patterns of restraint. In a single individual, therefore, one may see cyclic behavior: periods of inhibition, followed by periods of impulsive discharge, followed again by inhibition. This is the dynamic explanation for the relative prominence of behavior disorders in adolescence and the relative infrequency of specific psychiatric symptoms. It must be clear that this is an expression of the fluidity of both the self-system and the conscience in the adolescent personality, and the corresponding unreliability of the repressive mechanisms.

Of some relevance here is the adolescents' addiction to excitement and danger, the thrill of deliberately daring the powers of superior authority to catch and punish them for their excesses. In this behavior, they seek to measure their power against that of authority. They crave the satisfaction of outwitting and triumphing over authority, but beneath this façade always lurks the apprehension of the day of judgment. This type of motivation often finds expression in bizarre, irrational, and delinquent acts, such as walking a narrow roof ledge, stealing automobiles, etc.

Quantitatively viewed, the guilt related to sex drives and the corresponding aggression is often intense. In this connection, one important point must be made: Adolescents are not guilty about sex per se, but only as the release of the sexual urge is conceived as an act injurious to some other person. In the oedipal conflict, the guilt is not derived from the wish to possess the mother's love, but rather from the urge to inflict injury on the rival father. Because of the excessive nature of the guilt, a variety of defensive devices are brought into play in an effort to allay it. One means for evading conscious guilt is provided in the mechanism of "externalizing" conscience. This is a device for displacing responsibility to the person who personifies conscience. In essence, it implies "let so-and-so do the worrying for me." Still another device for dealing with guilt is the assumption of a defensively passive attitude. This is an effort to avoid responsibility for the initiative. "Let the other person do it first" is the means for shifting the burden of guilt. Another defense, closely related, is the avoidance of completion of an act which will incite guilt. The act may be begun, and it may be carried to near completion, but by magical thinking, so long as the act fails of actual completion, there need be no guilt.

This mechanism is conspicuously demonstrated in attitudes toward masturbation and sexual aggression. Masturbation and heterosexual behavior falling short of intercourse may be freely indulged, but guilt is avoided if the act falls a little short of completion. The concrete symbol of completion varies from one adolescent to the next. This trend of behavior is clearly exemplified in those cases where actual orgasm must be avoided at all costs, both in masturbation and in heterosexual play. Or, it may be demonstrated in cases of so-called "mental masturbation," where pleasure is experienced at a fantasy level but is not permitted in reality. Such adolescents may indulge in the wildest kind of sexual fantasies, may even experience orgasm, and yet may not permit themselves to touch the genital. An inevitable corollary of this defensive behavior is, of course, the incompleteness of the pleasure experienced. The measure of actual indulgence varies, but the sexual pleasure is never fulfilled. The feelings are numbed; boys may react with disappointment or disgust to masturbation and may suppress it altogether. In such instances, sometimes orgasm occurs without erection and often without pleasure. The girls may feel excitation close to orgasm, then experience a sudden and complete cessation of pleasurable feeling. In minor contacts with boys, the girls may say that kissing gives them no feeling whatever.

Illustration: A sixteen-year-old boy, the only child of two highly intelligent parents, was referred to the clinic allegedly because he was "adolescing too rapidly." His parents were especially alarmed one time when he shot off his father's hunting rifle right in their own home. They were also worried because he insisted on climbing across the ledge of the roof, "just for fun."

This boy was intellectually far advanced. He talked freely with his mother about his sexual preoccupations. In fact, she relished it. He was extremely close to his mother. She took an obvious pleasure in reliving his adolescent sexual experiences with him, kidded him about his wish to exhibit his penis to her, etc. At the same time, she was an alarmist, exaggerated his illnesses, encouraging him to nurse himself carefully with each cold.

This boy had no conscious worries about masturbation; indulged in it regularly, experienced intense pleasure in "mental masturbation," but felt completely numb if he attempted manual masturbation. Moreover, though he had masturbated for years, he was completely unable to carry it to the point of ejaculation. This changed only after he had been treated for some time. Firing his father's gun at home was a symbolic substitute act, indicative of his frustrated wish to experience actual ejaculation.

Adaptive Problems of Adolescence

When the quantity of guilt is large, there is a strong trend toward masochistic motivation. Sado-masochistic behavior is especially prominent in adolescence. The pleasure element may be mostly or entirely concealed, and in its place we see more the experiencing of suffering, which reflects the need for self-punishment. Sometimes the suffering clearly outweighs the pleasure; sometimes the pleasure is highly significant but is merely covered up by the more obvious suffering. Depending on the degree of guilt, and the basic character structure, one may see every variety of self-punishment: castration fantasies of all sorts, impotence, sterility, incapacitating fatigue, pain associated with menstruation and masturbation, fears of illness and death. To counteract such anxieties, there are compensatory fantasies of magical omnipotence, immunity to hurt, and immortality.

Illustration: A sixteen-year-old boy, referred to the clinic from school after taunting a female teacher with obscene drawings and lewd suggestions of intimacy. On examination, this boy was found to be suffering from acute, panicky fears of death which came on suddenly at night and horrified him to the point where he felt that he was losing his mind.

He is the only child of professional, middle-class parents; the father, a teacher; the mother, a social worker. As a child, he suffered from nightmares. For years he carried on an active fantasy life, in which he inflicted cruel sexual tortures on a loose type of woman, or rescued a pure, ideal type of woman from attack by other men and then himself had sexual relations with her. In these fantasies, he was always the hero. In his usual, everyday behavior, he was well controlled, respectful to his parents, coöperative. In his mind, women fell sharply into two groups: those like his mother, with whom he could have a real friendship, but with whom sex was completely excluded; and, in contrast, the sexually promiscuous type of woman, on whom he might freely release his sexual urges but whom he regarded as a low, dirty creature who inevitably made him feel a deep disgust with himself. He had an active social and athletic life, but basically was very lonely.

During his childhood, his mother was frequently out of the home, immersed in social welfare activities. Her attitude toward the patient was well meaning, but she had little real understanding of his needs. His father was naïve, and felt it to be his moral duty to warn the boy vigorously against masturbation and the dangers of venereal infection. Both parents were overzealous in their ambitions for this only child and extolled his virtues to the skies.

A frequent observation among adolescents is the tendency to dissociate temporarily the emotional expressions of hostility and sex. Hostile feeling and sexual drives become temporarily dissociated in the adolescent's relationship to his parents. Often the full hostility is directed against the parents, while the sexual needs are directed away from the parents, toward outside persons. Later, this defensive trend is reversed. When the adolescent's conflicts have subsided, and the hostility is less, the love interests revert to the parents.

Oedipal conflict of every shade is prominent in adolescence. The patterns of relationship to the parents which prevailed at the age of five or six years are reactivated. The emotional tendencies inherent in these relationships are affected now, however, by overt sexual pressures, and the increased maturity of the adolescent. The oedipal configuration rarely shows itself in pure, unadulterated form. Instead, its manifestations are heavily tinged with the influence of pregenital character traits. The partial components of the sexual drive are conditioned in their expression by the basic character structure. Incestuous fantasies are commonly present in adolescence, often just below the surface of consciousness, sometimes fully conscious. They often involve both the parent and sibling of the opposite sex. The content of the fantasy often discloses the specific parts of the parent's body to which the adolescent has a special attachment. This, in turn, illuminates the specific character of the repressed sexual urges, all highly patterned by the basic character patterns. The degree of oral dependent need and the degree of sadistic possessiveness which characterize the adolescent's attitude toward the parents are clearly reflected in the specific content of sexual fantasies.

The striving for a stable sexual identity, sensitively influenced by the vicissitudes of oedipal conflict, frequently reflects some degree of confusion. The partial identification with each parent results in some measure of bisexual identity, the boy having some feminine tendencies, the girl having some masculine tendencies. The so-called "inverted oedipal attachment" and unconscious

Adaptive Problems of Adolescence

homosexual leaning represent part of this same picture. Homosexual fear is much more common than is imagined. In this culture, in the process of maturation, some degree of injury to masculinity is common, and passive dependent tendencies in the male are reinforced. In the development of female children, the necessity for shifting the love interest from mother to father, and also the culturally conditioned competition between the sexes, tends to encourage in girls some degree of persistent dependence on mother figures, and envy of men. Attachments to persons of the same sex are used as a protection against the dangers of heterosexual intimacy. Thus, there is the tenacious clinging of girls to mother or girl friend, and the tendency of boys to form themselves into a mutually protective gang when they go seeking heterosexual adventures. The residual narcissism of adolescents also plays a significant role in the preservation of friendships with those of the same sex, and those most like themselves.

Illustration: A sixteen-year-old girl, confused, unstable, preoccupied with sexual fantasies, extremely intelligent but too disorganized to do satisfactory school work. Although a very attractive girl, she was unpopular with both sexes. Her social attitude was biting, spiteful, belligerently destructive.

She was absorbed with fantasies of being raped. She liked the idea of exciting boys sexually, but conceived of contacts with boys as a struggle for physical supremacy. She imagined wrestling or fist fights with boys; she seized all opportunities to humiliate members of the male sex. Beneath this aggression, she had an intense fear of being trapped in a dependent, submissive, childlike position in which she might be forced to confess defeat. Overtly, she was cocky, proud, boastful, and attempted to deny her fears. Underlying all this was a profound disillusionment in not being wanted or loved as a girl, and deep feelings of guilt and worthlessness.

She pretended to like her dominant role; pretended to enjoy to the fullest her tactics of revenge against males. Behind all this lurked a helpless child, weak, dependent, lonely, wishing she could trust someone enough to curl up in his arms and go to sleep. She did not dare surrender her vigilance, however, because of her fears of being hurt or being exploited sexually.

Having been reared in a sophisticated home, she had mild experiences of seduction at a young age with friends of her parents who were writers. She was overdependent on her mother, violently hated her father, but could not trust either parent. As children, she and her brother were often left for long periods with grandparents while the parents traveled.

We have here a strong tendency to social and sexual delinquency, based on primary emotional deprivation and confusion of sexual identity.

The anxiety and fear of punishment which adolescents feel about actual sexual intercourse is clearly demonstrated in their fantasies in another, though indirect, way. In daydreams, or in the so-called "wet dreams" of boys, coital relations are not usually carried to completion. Boys will frequently allege thoughts of intercourse, but close questioning usually reveals that the fantasy has stopped short of it. More often than not, in these fantasies the girls preserve the protection of their clothes, or some other symbolic barrier is interposed which effectively foils the desire for intercourse. Similar considerations hold for the waking and sleeping dreams of girls. Careful study of the dream content will disclose signs of anxiety and symbols of prohibition of the completed sex act. Closely related to this phenomenon is another tendency, holding much the same significance. Confused and contradictory concepts of sexual organs and functions may exist side by side in the mental life of adolescents. One set of concepts usually represents the unrealistic images of sex derived from childhood fantasy; the other set represents the more realistic, factual notions of sex obtained in later years. These two contradictory systems often carry on a parallel existence, occupying, in some adolescents, dissociated compartments of the mind. The infantile, distorted concepts of sex persist because they are protected from impact with reality. They continue to influence significantly the adolescent's behavior. In other adolescents, the contradictory concepts of sex clash openly, with the result that the adolescent is overtly confused.

The anxiety, which is activated by an awareness of the mature aspects of sex, impels the adolescent to cling to childhood notions which are less threatening to his defensive attitudes. Repression of sexual conflict in adolescence is extremely unstable, is never complete, and impels some degree of reliance on a variety of aux-

Adaptive Problems of Adolescence

iliary defenses against anxiety. This has obvious relevance for matters pertaining to sex education. Regrettably, sex education is not a simple procedure. Many of the superficial forms of sex education fail utterly and, at times, do more harm than good because information and advice are given without relation to the specific quality of the individual adolescent's defenses against sexual anxiety.

A few examples will illustrate: the adolescent who preserves the fantasy that his parents are too decent to indulge in the degrading experience of sexual relations, or if they have, it was only once or twice, for the purpose of having children; a girl who has been told repeatedly what sexual intercourse and childbirth are, but continues to have the fantasy that a girl who looks directly at a boy can be impregnated through the atmosphere; a boy whose mother deliberately exhibited herself to prove that the female genital differs from the male, but nevertheless preserves the fantasy that a woman has a penis.

From the foregoing discussions it must be quite clear that the sexual evolution of the adolescent and the resolution of identity conflict are tremendously influenced by the individual vicissitudes of past personality development. During the crucial changes of adolescence, the character traits established by past experience, the fixation points, and the regressive weaknesses of the individual clearly reveal themselves in their conditioning of the content and form of adolescent conflict and in their influence on social and sexual conduct.

Differential diagnosis in the adolescent era presents great difficulties. It is highly complicated by the infinitely changing façades of personality that are characteristic of this period. When is adolescent behavior, with its inevitable accompaniment of anxiety, conflict, confusion, and multicolored disturbances, "normal"? When is it "abnormal," and for what specific reasons?

During adolescence, anxiety, emotional confusion, erratic social behavior, shifting concepts of self and the outer world, weaknesses of reality perception, vacillating moral standards, instability and irregularity of impulse control, fickle, ambivalent interpersonal relations, may all be part of a normal, transitional adaptation. Transitory mild disturbance of these types may not constitute clinical pathology. Clinical diagnosis can in no way be based on intrinsic adolescent phenomena. Often, adolescent disturbance, per se, is mistakenly interpreted as representing clinical pathology, or per contra, actual psychiatric conditions are missed because they lie concealed behind the overlying façade of adolescent instability. How, then, to differentiate the abnormal? Accurate differential diagnosis is possible only when the subtle interplay of basic pathology and adolescent dynamics is clearly discerned. Specific forms of psychopathological illness underlie and subtly interact with the intrinsic adolescent phenomena. It is this dynamic relationship which must be disclosed by comprehensive examination. Correct appraisal of total personality function during adolescence requires close study in several dimensions: (1) current personality function; (2) past conditioning of personality; (3) pattern of movement of personality up to the present time; and (4) potential future course of personality, in a given life situation.

Accurate evaluation is possible only through a careful integration of knowledge of current personality function, with knowledge of genetic influences, from which is derived an evaluation of the pattern of movement of personality through current experience into adult patterns of integration.

The intrinsic phenomena of adolescence must be deeply understood in themselves, and in their over-all effect on basic character, so that behind this façade one can glimpse the underlying pathological trends. One needs always to bear in mind the manner in which a disposition to a specific psychiatric disability is affected by the intrinsic phenomena of adolescence. The task of diagnosis is complicated by the essential fluidity of adolescent personality which imparts relatively vague outlines to all psychiatric entities. In the final analysis, the test of the relative accuracy of clinical diagnosis is the ability to predict successfully the course of future behavior.

All aspects of this clinical study depend primarily on an exact and comprehensive examination of current personality function, which must include a careful assay of the role of surrounding cul-

Adaptive Problems of Adolescence

ture and group conditioning. Without exact appraisal of current behavior patterns, one cannot know clearly what one is trying to explain by way of genesis. The premature tendency to grope for genetic explanations, before achieving a correct formulation of present behavior, is one significant source of error in clinical judgments. With such blundering, one surely cannot visualize the path of future behavior.

Over a period of years, I have gradually evolved a guide for the evaluation of current personality function, which has proved quite useful.[1] The purpose of this outline is to provide a flexible guide for the examiner in achieving a more accurate appraisal of total personality function in the context of the present time and the present life situation. The scope of this outline is intentionally broad. It covers total personality organization, healthy functions as well as pathological formations. It is intended to illuminate both the assets and the liabilities of the individual. This form of diagnostic appraisal, to be used in close conjunction with the history, is considered to be important in establishing more clearly what is wrong with the patient's current adaptation and exactly what deviational behavior is to be treated.

The picture presented of the patient's personality should be live, unified, and dynamic, preserving the relatedness of the person to his immediate environment. Logically, the description should move from outside inward; that is, it should begin with a definition of the environment, and proceed from there to the "reactive" aspects of the patient's behavior, reflecting the patient's effort to adjust to that environment, and finally to a definition of the fixed, intrapsychic determinants of behavior which are relatively unmodified by environmental factors, and have been fixed by genetic causes. The last component of the evaluation provides the appropriate link with the psychoanalytically oriented history in which the emphasis is on genetic determination.

Such a guide can only be profitable if employed with discre-

[1] In formulating this guide, I have had helpful suggestions from the professional staffs of the Jewish Board of Guardians, Council Child Development Center, and the Psychoanalytic Clinic for Training and Research at Columbia University.

tion, with full flexibility, and with any modifications of content or emphasis that are needed to give a faithful portrayal of the uniqueness of the individual patient. Because of the ease with which such an outline can be misused, several precautions should be underlined:

1. The personality should not be dissociated from the environment.

2. The attention to detail and the effort to reach a more precise definition of component reactions should not result in atomization of the personality. The unity of the total personality must be preserved.

3. It is unnecessary to make statements covering every item of the outline—only those that are pertinent to the particular patient, and to the information available at a given time.

4. Since the outline is still imperfect, and there are some areas of overlapping, it is left to the discretion of the examiner to employ the guide in a useful manner, while at the same time minimizing the overlapping.

5. So far as possible, types of reaction should be illustrated with factual description rather than through surmise or speculation. In order best to accomplish this purpose, here and there examples of actual behavior may be given. Diagnostic and dynamic speculations should be clearly identified as such.

GUIDE FOR EVALUATION OF CURRENT PERSONALITY FUNCTION

Name: _____ Sex: _____ Status: _____
Age: _____ Race: _____ Occupation: _____
Intelligence: _____
Evaluation of environmental pattern: _____
Clinical diagnosis: _____ Character diagnosis: _____

I. GENERAL APPEARANCE AND BEHAVIOR:
Give a brief description of the patient as a living person; his attitudes, conduct, and general demeanor; also, where significant, the attitude toward the life situation and illness.

II. SYMPTOMS:
Enumerate the emotional disabilities, including a statement of the structured and unstructured symptoms, and any psychosomatic disorders that may be present.

III. The Environment of the Patient:
Give a concise statement of the significant environmental factors; the social, religious, and economic status, leading to a characterization of the cultural identity of the patient.

In addition, give a brief descriptive evaluation of the family configuration—the more significant relationships and the values which the family represents.

IV. Reality Adaptation:
Delineate those components of behavior which represent the patient's effort to adapt to his actual life situation.

In what directions is the effort successful, and in what directions does it fail? Bear in mind the patient's aspirations and goals and, where possible, indicate their relative adequacy.

What forms of reality are accepted?

What forms of reality are avoided, denied, or passively resisted?

What forms of reality are distorted, by what means? (Correlate this with later statement concerning defenses.)

V. Interpersonal Relations:
   A. Attitude toward others:
      1. Capacity for personal relationships
         a) Minimal capacity (infantile personality and extreme narcissism)
         b) Limited capacity (immature, "pregenital")
            (1) Dependent tendency
               (a) Passive dependent strivings—passive aggression ("oral character")
               (b) Tendency to deny dependent needs resulting in emotional detachment
            (2) Possession and control of other persons ("anal character")

            Characterize the ambivalence in these levels of relationship
         c) Mature capacity ("object" relationships)
            (1) With anxiety
               i) Identification with parents
               ii) Excessive submission
               iii) Excessive rebellion
               iv) Fear of punishment
            (2) Without anxiety
               i) Full achievement of individuality
               ii) Normal assertiveness
   B. Attitude toward self:
      1. Characterize the degree of self-absorption (egocentricity) and the degree of narcissism
      2. Characterize the patient's concept of self; his self-esteem, superiority, inferiority, his idea of self as a person, his inner image

of his own identity. Is the patient's image of his identity clear, unified, or dissociated and confused, etc.? (Use whatever descriptive terms seem to fit the patient's concept of self.)
3. Describe the idealized image of self toward which the patient aspires.
4. What discrepancy is there between the real concept of self and the idealized image?
5. What specific patterns of inferiority exist?
6. What trends toward compensatory self-aggrandizement are there?
7. What is the basis of the patient's confidence in specific areas of achievement? What patterns of self-condemnation and rejection in failure are found?
8. What are the patient's goals and the actual achievements? To what degree do they coincide and to what degree is there discrepancy?
9. Insight: What degree of real understanding does the patient have of his own function?

VI. QUALITY OF AFFECTS:
   A. Spontaneity ⎫
   B. Stability   ⎪
   C. Depth; richness ⎬ relation to activity pattern
   D. Appropriateness ⎪
   E. Flexibility ⎭
   F. Capacity for rapport
   G. Range of emotional interests
      1. Broad or constricted
      2. Genuine or pretended
      3. Lasting or temporary and fickle

VII. ANXIETY:
   A. Quantity
   B. Quality—acute, chronic, or intermittent; diffuse or organized in symptom formation; panic reactions (relate to patterns of control and defense)

VIII. INTEGRATION OF DRIVES:
   A. General integration; adequate or deficient; integration at levels of feeling, thought, and action
   B. Degree of impulsivity
      1. Conscious
      2. Unconscious
   C. Control of impulses at periphery of personality (i.e., suppression of action)
   D. Control of inner impulses; unconscious control (repression)
      1. Normal
      2. Deficient
      3. Excessive
   E. Capacity for pleasure and spontaneous self-expression
      1. Adequate

Adaptive Problems of Adolescence

      2. Deficient
      3. Conscience function excessive in quantity; deviant in quality
      4. Guilt tendency and guilt equivalents:
         a) Depression
         b) Suicidal tendency
         c) Other self-destructive patterns

IX. DEFENSE PATTERNS:
    A. Quality
      1. Range of defenses (narrow or wide)
      2. Rigid or changeable (shift from one defense to another)
      3. Reliability of defenses
      4. Panic reaction followed by emotional disorganization
    B. Types of defense (which used mainly?)
      1. Avoidance
      2. Opposition
      3. Substitution of aggression for anxiety
      4. Denial of external reality
      5. Denial of psychic reality; denial of elements of personal identity
      6. Repression
      7. Projection
      8. Introjection
      9. Displacement
      10. Condensation
      11. Compensation
      12. Reaction formation
      13. Rationalization
      14. Sublimation

X. CENTRAL CONFLICTS:
    A. Formulate the salient unconscious conflicts of the patient, as exemplified in the patient's symptoms, and in the disturbance in his relations with other persons.
    B. Correlate these conflicts with the type of anxiety and the main defenses which the patient uses to control his anxiety.
    C. Correlate these conflicts with the genetic patterns which represent their origin.
    D. Point emphasis to discrepancy between the contexts of conscious conflict and unconscious conflict.

Having made the evaluation of current personality function, it is in order to attempt to find answers to the following questions:

1. What part of the behavior represents intrinsic adolescent change?

2. What part represents the reaction to current environmental stimuli?

3. What part, if any, is constitutional?

4. What part is the product of fixed intrapsychic patterns conditioned by past life experience, especially the early family life?

5. How do the intrinsic adolescent phenomena influence the basic personality trends?

6. How do the basic personality trends influence the adolescent phenomena?

7. What is the probable future course of personality?

One caution should be borne in mind: a mere knowledge of unconscious tendencies in the individual, no matter how extensive, gives no clew to total personality function and, therefore, is insufficient for clinical diagnosis. For this, comprehensive knowledge of the patterns of total personality integration is necessary.

Now, a few comments regarding specific types of psychopathology: Adolescent instability may be a precipitating factor for any form of psychiatric disorder. There are, however, a few categories which merit special attention.

The one condition most clearly precipitated in adolescence is schizophrenia. The ego fragility, the weakness of repression, the inefficiency of defenses, the adolescent's closeness to his own unconscious, tend strongly to push into an overt state any latent schizophrenic trends. It is true that, in some instances, schizophrenia may become clinically manifest only in later years—in the third, fourth, and occasionally even the fifth decade—but when this occurs, the individual's fate, in the writer's opinion, has already been decided in adolescence, through the fixation during this stage of significant patterns of vulnerability.

Only occasionally is manic-depressive psychosis precipitated. Fairly commonly, psychoneurotic depressions break out in adolescence. Of considerable dynamic relevance in this connection is the deflection back on the self of hostility intended for the parents. Self-depreciatory trends are inevitably related to the adolescent's hostile wish to crush the idealized image of the parents. The occurrence of the classical forms of psychoneuroses, the so-called "transference neuroses," represent simply the reactivation of neurotic patterns, already evidenced in earlier years but now highly colored by the dynamic events of adolescence.

Adaptive Problems of Adolescence

Regardless of the type of pathology which emerges in adolescence, the typical symptoms of each psychiatric entity are significantly affected by the total dynamic movement characteristic of adolescence. It is, therefore, an imperative necessity to discern the course and ultimate destination of such movement. Without such discernment, reliable diagnosis is not possible.

Now then, how do these multiple and interlocking considerations pertain to the question of psychotherapy? Is adolescence a good or a bad time for treatment? This question has been productive of a highly interesting controversy. There are proponents on both sides of the fence. The fact is, however, that standards for the application of psychotherapeutic process in adolescence are less uniform than the standards of therapy for any other period of life. Historically viewed, guiding principles for the therapy of adults were the first to evolve; more recently, criteria for the treatment of children; but a consensus on basic principles for the treatment of adolescents has yet to be achieved.

There are some who claim that in adolescence the instability of the self-system, the erratic, unpredictable changes in social conduct, the acute anxiety over sexual tensions, tend seriously to hamper efforts at psychotherapy. There are others who emphasize the self-absorption and high narcissism of this period as deterrents to therapy; therefore, they counsel patience and argue for a postponement of therapy. The argument runs like this: "Wait till the peak of adolescent turbulence has passed; wait till the personality structure has congealed into its adult mold, when ego structure is more stable—then you can treat more effectively."

There are other therapists, however, who with equal conviction argue the other way. I count myself among these. I am convinced, on the basis of personal experience, that adolescence is an era strongly favorable for therapy. I believe that the very fluid qualities of adolescent dynamics, while constituting a potential danger to the success of therapy, may in the end, if correctly exploited, be advantageous for therapy. The adolescent personality, being dynamic and suggestible, is highly amenable to all external influence, including the therapeutic one.

In the beginning, certain factors may make the task of establishing rapport more difficult: the adolescent's characteristic mistrust of adults, his shift of allegiance to his peers, his egocentricity, evasiveness, and belligerence. I have found, often, that at the start the transference problems are touchy, delicate, and frequently quite complicated. Access to the adolescent's significant experience is difficult to achieve, and the flow of contact may be erratic. The adolescent's sense of responsibility to the therapeutic situation may be unsteady. Also, if the therapist does not prove himself worthy in the initial tests, and unintentially injures the patient's self-esteem, he may easily lose the patient. These are all serious potential risks for the therapy.

However, if the therapist skillfully pilots his way through these early dangers, the therapeutic tie becomes intensely strong, reliable, and is able to withstand even serious crises. In the later stages of therapy, adolescents show extraordinary powers for real working through of conflicted emotions; they have unusual capacities for psychic perception and for accumulation of new insight into unconscious process. Once past the early hazards of the therapeutic relationship, it is my experience that adolescents become excellent patients and benefit enormously.

For selected cases, depth analysis works exceedingly well. I make this statement with some qualifications; the analytic technique must be carefully adapted in specific ways to individual adolescent need. Since the patient's reality-testing capacities are often inadequate, the therapist must definitively personify social reality for the patient. Wherever the ego orientation proves defective, the therapist should be ready and able to translate reality for the patient in a simple, easily assimilable, and unthreatening way. This is vital to the adolescent's effort to build an integrated control over his emotional drives.

Therapy should be conducted on an easy, flexible, informal basis, making the adolescent as comfortable as possible, and allowing the broadest possible range of adaptation to rapid changes in situation and behavior. The therapist must assume a strongly supporting role; he is required, by the adolescent's need, to be a direct parent substitute. Through the feeling of protection which the adolescent derives from this relationship, he is encouraged to face the anxiety which he feels in expanding experiences and relationships. It is important for the therapist continuously to counteract potential threats of injury to the patient's self-esteem, and thus carefully guard the adolescent's sense of individuality.

Of particular importance is the working out of the confusion and anxiety which are associated with the patient's striving for a more secure sexual identity. In this struggle, the adolescent requires sustained help in achieving adequate control over his sexual urges and the associated aggression. Frequently, a patient is excessively preoccupied with sexual need, but is completely unready for sexual experience, due to specific emotional distortions and generalized immaturity. It is the therapist's function, in such situations, to help the patient clearly to see his unreadiness, and through this to win the patient's coöperation in waiting until the time is ripe. Often such patients are materially relieved by being directly told that they are not yet prepared for such realities.

The issue of the therapist's identification with the patient is, of course, of central significance. The patient sorely needs the feeling that the therapist is on his side, feels his emotional pain; but empathy must be controlled and regulated by the necessary insights.

Mention was made earlier of the caseworker's therapeutic aptitude with adolescents. Here we have a fusion, in a single person, of two advantageous factors: a young person who symbolizes a peer or a "big brother" or "sister," an ally in the struggle with authority, and a person equipped with professional skills. The capacity for empathy is a decided asset, provided the caseworker has, himself, weathered the adolescent storm, achieved a workable reintegration of personality, and built up the emotional resources indispensable to a correct application of insight. On occasion, a worker fails to make the most of his capacity for empathy because of a lack of confidence in his own mastery of adolescent conflicts. Sometimes, in place of true empathy, the worker indulges in unconscious projection, with unfavorable results. Thus, a young worker, deficient in emotional integration, may falter and fail in therapy with an adolescent.

In recent years, I have experienced a real advantage in supplementing individual psychotherapy with group psychotherapy. The group experience has special value in the context of the adolescent need for an exchange of experience with his peers. This level of therapeutic influence, that is, working out conflicts in coöperation with other adolescents, is irreplaceable.

Adolescence—Its Implications for Family and Community

VIOLA W. BERNARD, M.D.

PREVENTIVE PSYCHIATRY is rapidly emerging as an urgent national mental health necessity as the staggering incidence of mental illness and emotional maladjustment is being recognized. The adolescent phase of development represents a juncture crucial for later mental health. As such it properly becomes a major public health challenge and responsibility.

We have come to regard adolescence as a phase of maturation which is induced basically by biological change, entails profound interaction between the individual adolescent personality and his surrounding culture, is largely shaped by the adolescent's past personality development, and lastingly influences all categories of subsequent personality adjustment. It follows, then, that the degree of childhood developmental health, the ways he meets the adaptive tasks of adolescence, and the kind of world the adolescent must live in constitute a triple set of considerations governing the main directions of mental hygiene approach.

Much more is known about the personality aspect of child development than is actually practiced. Everything conducive to optimum adjustment of children can be regarded as preventive psychiatry in relation to adolescence. This is certainly not an occasion for a review of child psychology, but it may be pertinent to attack some existent compartmentalizing whereby health and welfare needs of children, adolescents and adults are dealt with separately with obsolete disregard for our modern knowledge of the implications of genetic continuity. Thus, in a sense, what the family and community do, or do not do, for its children is highly relevant to what kind of adolescents those children become.

One way to help many adolescent children would be to provide more adequate facilities of proven need and value in their early years. For example, there is no kindergarten space for 10,000 children, in the city of New York, despite some recently added classes. Properly staffed day care facilities and nursery schools are of demonstrated importance in family life. New York has far too few, and those are in jeopardy. Child health stations serving preschool children and their mothers are strategic opportunities for preventive psychiatry, but except for a few sporadic demonstrations, New York City's health stations are not equipped to provide this service. Parents are eager for expert information about infants' care and can often better accept it in such a setting. The staffing of such health stations with clinical personnel trained in the newer concepts of child development is needed.

Another discrepancy between knowledge and practice is seen in the lack of facilities for the early treatment of emotionally disturbed children of preschool age. A start has been made by the establishment in New York of the Council Child Development Center. In Detroit, the Cornelia Corner, an organization of psychiatrists, obstetricians, pediatricians, and social workers, illustrates a type of coöperation in safeguarding psychological health at the outset of life. The family agency's role in helping family life provides another valuable means of carrying out this needed function.

How the community copes with the needs of its neglected, dependent, disturbed, handicapped, and early delinquent children has great bearing on how those children experience the added pressures of their adolescence. We know too that the kind of elementary school experience that the community provides is vitally related to the child's preparation for adolescence. But Dr. William C. Menninger recently reported that 2,000,000 children throughout the country between the ages of six and fifteen were not in any kind of school in 1940.

My purpose in briefly citing these areas of community services for child conservation—and there are many more—is to emphasize their prophylactic relevance to adolescent and adult mental health.

Implications of Adolescence

Any and all measures for assisting the constructive outcome of the adolescent period of transition constitute preventive psychiatry in terms of later life. Since the adolescent is still dependent on family, but centering more and more of his life in the wider community, both family and community can contribute significantly by omission and commission to the successful outcome of the adolescent's adaptive tasks. These have been described by Lawrence Frank and others, as:

1. Becoming independent and self-directing, progressively emancipated from dependence upon the family and from the submissive obedience to their commands
2. Clarifying and accepting the masculine or feminine role and learning the appropriate conduct, feelings and patterns of relationships
3. Establishing his or her place in social life, developing relations to the many different agencies and institutions, proving one's adequacy
4. Revising one's image of the self and adjusting one's childhood beliefs to the activities of social life and adjusting one's aspirations to the goals and values by which the individual directs his life career.

The ever present dynamic interaction between every individual and his culture is dramatically heightened in the adolescent. The pace and turbulence of present social change, productive of a sense of chaos, are doubly hard on adolescents because of the accelerated inner changes they undergo. The degree of success we achieve or fail to achieve in working out the broad social problems of the day directly affects the stability of our young people. Direct and indirect effects of the recent war and the threat of another, the American dilemma between democratic ideals of equality and the social imperative to succeed by ruthless competitive aggression, discrimination against minority groups and its effect both on victims and on aggressors, serve to stimulate still greater confusion and anxiety in youngsters grappling with the insecurities of establishing a changing self and a changing role in a changing world.

The cultural discrepancy between both the moral and legal codes of sexual behavior and actual sexual practices profoundly complicates psychosexual development and conflicts. The Kinsey report on male sexual behavior impressively documents the inconsistencies between our sex laws, written and unwritten, and sexual facts. One of his findings of significance to our topic is that late adolescence is the period of greatest male sexual activity, rather than the twenties and thirties as so often supposed. By sexual activity is meant a variety of experiences culminating in sexual climax. Masturbation, nocturnal emission, and heterosexual petting, without intercourse, are therefore, included in this total of adolescent sex activity.

The systems of social rank and status-stratified classes in this country present added major difficulties to the socialization process for many of the nation's adolescents. As Allison Davis has pointed out: "To make low-status children anxious to work hard, study hard, save their money and accept stricter sex mores, our society must convince them of the reality of the rewards at the end of the anxiety-laden climb."

The vulnerability of the adolescent period imposes a responsibility on both the family and larger community. A few considerations regarding treatment of the more troubled adolescents seem appropriate to the more effective discharging of that responsibility.

My own experience supports the conclusion "adolescence is an era strongly favorable for therapy." The characteristic state of flux renders the individual highly susceptible to new experiences and influences. This offers an opportunity for the insertion of needed elements into the growth process itself as the personality reorganizes into the more solid structure of adulthood. Therefore, the nature of the experiences and influences can be uniquely decisive in the reinforcement or constructive resolution of whatever latent psychopathology the adolescent brings with him from his total earlier development. Expanding insight into the dynamics of the adolescent process permits modification of therapeutic principles and techniques to fit adolescent needs. As an in-between phase of maturation it demands a brand of specialized help of its own, rather than merely carried-over procedures from child or adult psychiatry. As Caroline Zachry has

Implications of Adolescence

stated: "Therapeutic techniques are geared to the fact that he [the adolescent] is neither man nor child but both."

An elastic concept of therapy includes many varieties of assistance, differing in level, goal, point of emphasis and method of approach. Help may be offered indirectly, as through improvement of the social climate of a high school class, or directly, ranging from relatively simple reassurance and guidance to intensive, analytic psychotherapy.

One may generalize that the help given to adolescents should be in ways of enabling their own efforts at working out solutions. While this is a principle of all therapy, it is more apt to be disregarded, and yet it is of special importance to adolescents. It is frequently overlooked because the youngsters often appear to be so helpless and floundering that various mixtures of authoritative and protective impulses are aroused in the helping adults. The importance, however, is twofold: in the establishment of rapport, because of the sensitivity to coercion; and in the nature of the assistance, which must not play into the strong regressive temptation to evade independence. The choice of approach, of course, should be dictated by the youngster's needs and available avenues of access.

The typical dependent-independent conflict must be taken into account as one of the frequent resistant obstacles presented by youngsters. This dilemma may be solved often if the adolescent shares in choosing the remedial regime, thus satisfying the emancipation urge. Within the framework of his own freedom of choice he can then better afford to accept imposed limitations on freedom, with lessened arousal of defensive revolt, while gratifying the need for impulse control, reduction of guilt, and ego strengthening.

For example, a fifteen-year-old girl of wealthy background, attending an excellent boarding school, failed academically, displayed antisocial behavior, despite patient, understanding attempts by the school staff, and was finally expelled for stealing. The school had been chosen by her neurotically maladjusted, rejecting, divorced parents for whom the girl's social and academic success was largely tied up with their own prestige. By failing, the youngster was punishing her parents, although in a self-destructive way, with attendant feelings of increased guilt, inadequacy and general unhappiness. She flatly refused the urging of her parents that she see the psychiatrist, who must have seemed to her but another extension of hated and feared parental control.

After her expulsion, however, both parents gave up in angry disgust. This form of rejection was easier to take than the previous form, disguised as parental concern. Freed of their domination, she floundered around for a bit and then, by her own initiative, discovered a work-school which she insisted on attending. The parents were inclined to refuse, but were prevailed upon by the psychiatrist, who recognized the girl's needs that were determining the selection, as well as the value to her of making her own choice. Here the psychiatrist's role was indirect via consultation with the parents.

She made a spendid record in the school of her choice, academically and socially. The parents were amazed at her enthusiastic adherence to the exacting, rigid routine and discipline. The school is run along coöperative work lines, the youngsters putting in long hours between their academic requirements and work responsibilities. Standards are high, slackness is not tolerated, and penalties are readily imposed for poor performance. The student group cohesiveness was great, however, and loyalty to the school intense, with the feeling that the school staff was strict, but fair. So seriously did the youngsters take their responsibilities that most of them voluntarily returned to school ahead of time at the end of the Christmas vacation, lest their jobs suffer. This girl had found for herself a sense of belonging and a feeling of being needed, in exchange for which she could accept standards of conduct and limitation of impulse-gratifying, welcoming them, in fact, as external supports for her own inadequate ego equipment. Had she not chosen this school herself, she probably would have reacted rebelliously and failed to use the therapeutic ingredients available there. The strengthening effect of this experience, it is hoped, will help to bring about gradual reduction of her reliance on such external support of conscience and greater assumption of her capacity to internalize her self-direction. Over-prolongation of such an environment could lead into her under-

Implications of Adolescence

development, just as had the earlier insufficiency of such external ego support.

Sensitive timing in the introduction and withdrawal of elements needed for growth and the exertion of various types of pressure toward adult functioning, in dosage commensurate with the rapidly shifting stages of the adolescent, is essential to effective therapy with that age group. This therapeutic principle is illustrated by an eighteen-year-old girl whose early months of casework therapy were largely dominated by an exaggerated, overt attitude of rebellious independence. This also characterized her acting out, both within and outside the therapeutic situation.

When the time was ripe, in the clinical judgment of the caseworker and the consultant psychiatrist, the worker offered some interpretation concerning an essential area of highly charged emotional conflict underlying this girl's disturbance. She responded violently and stated her intention to break off treatment. Her reaction was skillfully handled by the worker, and the therapeutic value of the session was borne out when she returned for her next interview, which included, in addition, a significant shift in the symptomatic revolt to which we have already referred. The girl told the worker that she had been reviewing the year in her own mind and had come to the conclusion that when she had come to the worker, although she thought what she wanted was independence, she had not actually been ready for it and had been fooling herself in thinking that she was. She realized that although she acted and talked as though she were independent, she had actually relied on the worker to pull her through. She had not supported herself, gone to school, or held a job. She honestly did not believe that she could go to school and work part time. She had come to the conclusion that she would like to go to college, which was something toward which she had previously expressed disinterest. She asked the worker's help in a plan whereby she would be accepting financial help while attending school until the summer when she would seek a job with the intention of entering college in the fall and working her way through. She thought that for some people her age, asking for and accepting help now would be a backward step but that for her it was a forward step to recognize her real dependence, to accept it, and use it as a means to becoming really independent in the future. The worker agreed and went along with the plan.

Thus, during the course of direct treatment of adolescents, one must keep pace with a constant shifting and progression in the relative proportions of opposing needs and the various ways of meeting them. At a given period the youngster may need to rely more exclusively on the group of age mates and may seem to relegate the adult therapist to a relatively subordinate position as a defense. For almost a year a sixteen-year-old patient could only report her dreams to the analyst after they had been first confided to, and talked over with, her circle of friends. As Caroline Tryon puts it: "It is in this group that by doing they learn about the social process of our culture. They clarify their sex roles by acting and being responded to, they learn competition, coöperation, social skills, values and purposes by sharing a common life." [1]

Somewhat later, however, the group allegiance may diminish in favor of the next type of relationship experience. Thus, one seventeen-year-old predelinquent explained after six months of casework therapy that she now felt that she had secured as much as she could use of what she needed from her crowd. She also felt that she had been able to give something to them. This was an experience that was necessary and helpful at a particular stage of her life, but she thought that it was no longer essential to her. This girl had desperately utilized her group of friends, not only for the purposes common to her age period, but as an almost total substitute for her home, with which she was in open revolt. In this instance, as in so many adolescent delinquents, the child-parent relation had been so disturbed throughout the successive stages of the girl's development that her teen-age break with home meant a more complete repudiation, with less acceptable past identifications to fall back on, and, therefore, greater weakness of personality structure than that of the youngster whose revolt is a transitional maneuver to establish a new position in relation

---

[1] Caroline M. Tryon, "Adolescent Peer Culture," in *Forty-third Yearbook of the National Society for the Study of Education*, Part II, "Adolescence" (Chicago: University of Chicago Press, 1944), p. 217.

Implications of Adolescence

to family and society and who uses the group as an intermediate source of strength to accomplish this. Depending on the degree of earlier disturbed child-parent relationships, the adolescent individual may use the new strengths and opportunities of growth to attempt a total demolishing overthrow of the family and its internalized elements within the self, as in the more disturbed adolescents, while in the so-called "normal" adolescents, the emancipation process, though involving revolt, is essentially the building of new extensions of personality on more or less self-accepted foundations of the previous self. More therapeutic rebuilding is obviously necessary, the less healthy or usable this earlier foundation. In seeking not only new, but old answers from the group, which the family failed to provide, the youngster, in turn, may feel at such a disadvantage with the group that she seeks out some adult whom she feels she can trust. Rather than a parent figure, however, the adolescent strives to choose an adult who, by one means or another, can fulfill a less threatening and conflicted image, such as that of older brother or sister, more experienced friend, or teacher, all of whom sidestep some of the threatening implications of the early parental image.

A girl whose family utterly failed her in meeting the essential needs of childhood and adolescence reacted with conduct disturbances and neurotic symptoms, for which she received help in a therapeutically conditioned environment, combined with some individual psychotherapy. Now, some years later, at nineteen and a college sophomore, she writes to the psychiatrist:

As to whether I would need psychiatric help now, I don't think I need it. My chief problem is to get a lot of questions answered. I feel I have much better insight now than I ever had before. My immediate problem is what is the proper conduct for me when out with the opposite sex. This is not in terms of Emily Post, but necking. Actually I have never had an opportunity to ask anyone as to what I think society expects of me and what is the accepted practice. I have finally got around to wanting to ask you about necking and other questions.

The letter was signed "Your friend, Ruth."

It is clear that this youngster needed to dissociate the therapist from the threatening connotations of "psychiatrist," which she rejects, in order to secure the needed help through the more acceptable channel of friendship, yet her inner perception of psychiatric need, if protected against the label, was demonstrated by her feeling unable to obtain answers to her pressing problems from anyone else. It may often be clinically advisable, as in this instance, that the psychiatrist or caseworker respect such a defense, at least at first, as a requisite condition for giving the needed help.

Available knowledge of the needs of adolescents and the ability to formulate their problems is far ahead of the application of such knowledge. Further research should and will go forward, but the community needs arousal from its apathy in providing for its young people.

Facilities for disturbed adolescents are deplorably insufficient and often unsuited to their purpose. And yet we know the gravity of neglecting such disturbances as well as the human salvage often possible by timely intervention during this period. Over-all planning is urgently needed in mapping out the various types of facility that should be available as coördinated services for adolescents. A referral service is valueless unless there are treatment resources to accept referrals. Careful diagnostic work-ups are futile and extravagant if there are no ways and means of carrying out recommendations. Unless the community provides itself with a comprehensive program for treating disturbed adolescents, it is questionable how much any component unit can accomplish other than research and demonstration.

Perhaps one reason for this state of affairs lies in a lack of agreement about the special nature of adolescents, thus fitting them, or perhaps "misfitting" them, into existent facilities developed for adults. Thus, adolescents committed to New York State hospitals, with a very few exceptions, are on the adult wards. Statistics in the New York State *Year Book for Mental Hygiene,* for instance, are not even broken down to indicate how many adolescents are hospitalized. It seems to me that this runs counter to all we have learned about the unique features of adolescence.

Sylvan Keiser has reported on a group of schizophrenia-like

Implications of Adolescence

reactions at puberty and regards them as benign psychopathological reactions of the adolescent period, mistakenly diagnosed as schizophrenia. He regards them as reactive states dependent on the recrudescence of infantile conflicts occurring during adolescence. His report is cited to emphasize the well-known difficulty of accurate differential diagnosis during adolescence. Scattered experience indicates the therapeutic advantage of separate adolescent psychiatric wards in city or state hospitals, equipped with school facilities related to the treatment program, and staffed with specially trained personnel. For years Bellevue Hospital had New York City's only psychiatric adolescent ward for boys, while the girls were put with adults. Two psychiatric wards for adolescents have finally been opened at Kings County Hospital, with twenty beds for boys and ten for girls, to service the boroughs of Brooklyn and Queens. Neither ward has any school facilities. Rockland State Hospital has a thirty-three-bed ward for disturbed adolescent boys. They have no school facilities, though some tutoring is available. Kings Park State Hospital has a children's ward for ages six to fourteen, for whom the care is primarily custodial rather than an active therapeutic program. No schooling is available, and occupational therapy is the only learning activity. Above the age of fourteen, the youngsters are with the adults. In the other New York State hospitals, adolescents are placed with the adult psychiatric patients.

It would appear that we have too little and the wrong kind of facility for the adolescent who is in need of psychiatric hospitalization, either for observation or for prolonged treatment. Further study is needed for an accounting of the numbers of children in this community who need such care, as well as what modifications may be needed in the type of mental hospital that is designed for adults. A frequently met and seldom solved problem is where to send a seriously disturbed adolescent who is too sick to stay home or at school, who cannot adjust in the usual children's institution, and who needs treatment in a controlled environment. I share the view of those who feel that we need some new kind of treatment facility for such youngsters—not exactly a mental hospital, school, or psychiatrically oriented institution, but yet something of all three.

The general shortage of psychiatrists and psychiatric clinics, of course, affects those adolescents who need and can accept psychotherapy. The Bureau of Child Guidance of the New York City Board of Education gives child guidance service to some of the city's high schools. The full time of three social workers and three psychologists, as well as part of the time of two psychiatrists, is assigned to the high school division. The budget allows for one more social worker and one more psychologist, whose positions have not yet been filled. When we consider that the total population of the city's high schools is 232,628, the amount of service in proportion to need is ridiculously low. It is interesting that the students in schools covered in this way are learning to refer themselves, indicating a need for help which the worker can usually meet only by attempting further referral, which is apt to be a frustrating experience because of the lack of treatment resources.

Many adolescents, for whom psychiatrists seem far too threatening, can accept casework help. The parent also is often opposed to psychiatric help for the youngster but can accept help from the children's or family agency. Gordon Hamilton has ably described psychotherapy of adolescents by social workers at the Jewish Board of Guardians, in her recent book.[2] She regards psychotherapy as a legitimate and appropriate specialization within the larger field of social work. Caseworkers at that agency, who receive specialized training as psychotherapists, work in continuous collaboration with staff psychiatrists.

Some disturbed adolescents, with various mixtures of conduct and neurotic disorders and difficult family situations, can use direct treatment only in combination with environmental changes. A therapeutically conditioned environment as a treatment setting has won its vital place in the therapeutic armamentarium for adolescents. A monograph published by the Jewish Board of Guardians [3] describes such an integrated use of total

[2] Gordon Hamilton, *Psychotherapy in Child Guidance* (New York: Columbia University Press, 1947).

[3] *Conditioned Environment in Case Work Treatment* (New York: Jewish Board of Guardians, 1944).

Implications of Adolescence

environment geared to the basic needs of adolescents in general and the special treatment requirements of the particular disturbed boys and girls comprising their groups. Leontine Young,[4] in reporting on another such project (fifteen adolescent girls at Wallkill Cottage), confirms earlier remarks on how one lack of resource may nullify the work of another. Thus, Miss Young describes setbacks in gains accomplished largely for lack of club-type residences in New York City where the girls could go after leaving the cottage, as an intermediate experience prior to assuming complete independence in their living arrangements. The Community Service Society has been developing a new resource for disturbed adolescents in the form of a diagnostic study home for girls who are receiving casework therapy at the agency.[5] Here again, the over-all facilities for this age group is such that some girls are kept on longer than is clinically indicated and others lose ground by resorting to undesirable living situations for lack of appropriate alternatives.

One valuable treatment feature of the therapeutically oriented environment for maladjusted adolescents—whether it be institution, boarding school, or study home—is the opportunity for "on-the-spot" therapy, as symptomatic behavior and relationship patterns manifest themselves in day-to-day living situations. For many adolescents—not only those in special environments—formal psychotherapy in an office interview at regular appointments arouses too much resistance to be tolerated, whereas the informal, spontaneous explanation, utilizing a kind of living out, as well as talking out, and arising in a natural setting, is often seized upon and assimilated. The natural setting may well be classroom, social club, athletic field, or "bull session." Group leaders, school guidance counselors, and teachers with some training and feeling for the understanding of behavior can be of great help in this way with the problems of the so-called "normal"

---

[4] Leontine R. Young, *The Treatment of Adolescent Girls in an Institution* (New York: Child Welfare League of America, Inc., 1945).

[5] Aileen C. Burton, Judith Katz Wallerstein, and Viola W. Bernard, "An Experimental Study and Treatment Home for Adolescent Girls under Casework Treatment," paper read at the annual meeting of the American Orthopsychiatric Association, April 13, 1948.

adolescent. Peter Blos emphasizes the advantages of the natural setting for offering psychological counseling to college students. Not only does the intramural setting enable the counselor to catch problems early and thereby accomplish more preventive results, but, as he says:

> Wherever such services are made part of a medical office or a student health service (which is primarily for physical attention), a psychological barrier is erected which tends to eliminate those cases which could profit most from psychological counseling. In addition, it must be recognized that referral to clinic or psychiatrist is for the college a drastic step, and for the student a frightening one. No one in any educational institution will take the responsibility for it except where the need is obvious.[6]

Dr. Blos limited his counseling to students with mild dysfunctions; those who needed intensive psychotherapy were referred for treatment.

I have said little about the school's role in the adolescent's adjustment process, perhaps because it is so vast and so important. Early spotting of danger signals and prompt attention to them, either within or outside the school, is, of course, one vital function from the mental hygiene aspect. The school nurse and physician may often recognize a trouble area and clear it up with appropriate reassurance, particularly in connection with the many fears of somatic deviations. School social workers, bridging home, school, and community resources in relation to the individual youngster's needs, should be in every school, especially in the more socially deprived areas of a city. Over and above these special services, in affecting the whole adolescent school population, is the social climate of the school which represents such a large part of each day's world to the student. A friendly or a hostile human atmosphere sets the tone of a school and influences the kind of learning, both academic and social, in addition to the essential teaching skills and curriculum content. The more totally an adolescent rejects his family and the identifications therein, the more exaggerated will be his dependence on the group for security, affection, and the acquisition of values and standards. Schools

[6] Peter Blos, "Psychological Counselling of College Students," *American Journal of Orthopsychiatry*, XVI, No. 4 (October, 1946), 571.

Implications of Adolescence

constitute a major experience of adolescent group life, and recent advances in the theoretical understanding of group dynamics may increasingly shed light on the teacher's role and its implications, as well as on many other aspects of the interactions of the group members. Fritz Redl, for example, has contributed significantly to some of the implications of group behavior in school and among juvenile delinquents. Kurt Lewin and his associates, in one of their many fascinating and pioneering studies in group dynamics, experimentally created varieties of social climate and found that the children who had an autocratic leader became much more aggressive, not toward the leader, but toward each other, using scapegoat mechanisms in contrast to the group with a democratic leader. Further investigations into group dynamics and group therapy offer perhaps one of the most promising areas of research in regard to adolescence.

Since adolescence involves an upheaval in relationship to parents, it follows that the adolescence of their children represents something of a vulnerable phase in the parents' life experience. Reciprocal drastic adjustments on the part of parents are abruptly demanded by the changes the youngsters undergo. The effect on parents, as in the case of the adolescents themselves, may vary from the "normal" degree of upset to profound disturbance, largely depending on the basic maturity of the parents.

Today's parents are yesterday's adolescents whose mode of working through that stage affects how they accomplish the current reversal of roles in the family drama. Having once centered so much hostility, fear, guilt, envy, desire and emotional conflict on their own parents during adolescence, the experience of the parental side of the interchange is, for many parents, unsettling to say the least.

Understanding the nature of the adolescent process provides one of the best methods for mitigating parental unhappiness and bewilderment. By understanding the youngster's need to belittle and defy as part of a developmental struggle rather than as primarily a personally directed loss of love, parents can weather the storm with greater emotional intactness, and also are less driven to retaliative hostility, which can set up a destructive cycle and imperil the outcome for the youngster. Popular dissemination of facts about adolescent behavior can be very helpful toward the gaining of such understanding by many normally secure parents. For instance, the realization of how variable is the age of onset and rate of growth of physical pubertal changes can be enormously reassuring. Likewise, many parents suffer undue alarm by failing to recognize the normalcy of emotional and behavioral deviations, while others neglect danger signals because of a false complacency. When the ignorance is more largely based on dearth of facts than on the need not to see them, various forms of factual parental education can be extremely helpful.

It has been repeatedly stressed that psychologically, adolescence constitutes, at least in part, a recrudescence of the individual's oedipal stage of childhood development. Perhaps there has been some insufficient recognition that the process of puberty in a child may serve to stimulate in the mother and father a reactivation of their own adolescence. Many of the parents' attitudes and emotional responses to their child may stem from this. Latent weaknesses and neurotic elements in the adult's adaptive development may come to the fore as the parent relives his past crucial life experience in the dual capacity of parent and child. The degree of unconscious neurotic involvement underlying the parental response to the adolescent child significantly influences the ultimate adjustment of both. For instance, counteroedipal and counterhostile reactions in the mother or father, interlocking with the youngster's oedipal pattern, may tip the balance against a successful resolution. An example is seen in the study of the family interrelationships of adolescent unmarried mothers. In many cases the illegitimate pregnancy is the outcome of a symbolic, unconscious acting out of the girl's Oedipus conflict. The girl's father, in many such cases, exhibits insufficiently repressed counteroedipal response to the maturing of his daughter. Although the seductive element in the relation may frequently be recognized, despite varying degrees of repressive disguise, the defensive side of the father's conflict often characterizes his conspicuous overt attitude, such as excessive punitive prohibitions against the usual adolescent boy-girl activities.

Implications of Adolescence

Another version may occur in homes where there is only one parent, through the death or separation of the other. The parent is then often unconsciously prone to substitute an adolescent son or daughter for the missing marriage partner. Such a parental need coincides with so many of the adolescent's inner temptations that it may prove a rather durable barrier against his ever achieving the emancipation essential to emotional maturity. By prematurely treating the youngster as an adult, and thus seemingly, on the surface, accelerating his adulthood, such a parent may actually fixate the youngster and effectively block his maturity. Examples of this may be seen among some of the middle-aged single women who much preferred to keep house for father, and the middle-aged bachelor for whom marriage, representing an attempted replacement of mother, as well as a freeing from her, is sought only after her death.

The same is true for the less directly psychosexual areas of conflict. Parents may be driven to excessive suppressive attacks against the adolescent through feeling overthreatened by the child's hostility, which they may unconsciously interpret in terms of their own former adolescent, repressed, aggressive violence against their own parents. Thus, a son's normal assertion of independence may touch off the father's repressed hatred of his own father, inducing irrational terror and counterattack against the boy.

Sometimes the youngster seems to offer an emotional opportunity to the parent for vicariously reliving a lost youthfulness. This can lead to an inconsistent and vacillating attitude, which for an adolescent is one of the most harmful. A mother may vacillate between tempting the daughter to fulfill prohibited urges of her own adolescence, only to turn around and discipline her with exaggerated parental severity, thus re-enacting her old impulse-conscience conflict at the expense of her daughter. This, in turn, augments the girl's hostility to her mother, seeming to confirm her sense of maternal unfairness accumulated throughout her life, and interacting with the reinforcing elements common to adolescence. It also leads into her need of projection of external blame, thus making it harder for her to face her own inner conflicts. For instance, a certain mother encourages her daughter in extravagant clothes-buying, clearly reliving her own wishful girlhood thereby, but then whips up the father's fury against the girl for exceeding her allowance, siding with the father in punishing her for her greedy transgression of his prohibitions and her irresponsibility with money. Unconsciously, this mother not only identifies with the girl in the clothes-buying sprees, but is jealous of her and needs to discredit her with the father.

The maturation of their children entails understandable threats for many parents, to which they react by various forms of opposition to the growing up. A wide diversity of parental needs and reaction patterns may thus be involved. The child's dependency may so serve the parents' needs that they have great difficulty in relinquishing a benevolent tyranny, which is often rationalized as loving protectiveness. The youngster's drive for self-direction may stimulate intensified parental hanging-on for fear of losing the child. Sometimes feelings of inadequacy, rivalry and suppressive hostility are aroused as the young emerging adult seems to present a competitive challenge, an unmistakable reminder of their own advancing years.

Thus, an insecure father may be jealous of his son's vigor, or a mother, fearful of the implications of her involution period, may be threatened by her daughter's good looks. This may account for such patterns of behavior as mothers who represent their daughters' age as much younger than is actually so and who make the youngsters dress as younger children as long as possible, in a futile attempt to prevent their development. Others may attempt an adjustment by relinquishing the mother role in favor of a sister relation. To the daughter this can mean the double hardship of maternal loss and rivalrous encroachment on her girlhood.

Not too infrequently, otherwise unsatisfactory marriages are long held together by the bond of children. Their growing up may precipitate the latent strains between husband and wife into more overt discord or separation. To illustrate: an eighteen-year-old son's leaving home for college served as a trigger to initiate a sequence of events culminating in the divorce of his parents. The mother had unconsciously compensated through her attachment to the son for the dissatisfactions with her husband. She had incompletely accepted her adult role, but had perpetuated a wishful sense of herself as a young girl. The value she derived from this fantasy was threatened simultaneously by the puberty of her daughter and the advent of her fortieth birthday about the time the boy left home. She could not face the actuality of maturity and was impelled into an impulsive love affair with a much younger man, who served to reaffirm her youthful attractiveness, substitute for her son, free her from her husband, and triumph over the upthrusting femininity of her daughter.

The adolescent may impel the parents to exploit the youngster's need for independence by denying his equally strong dependent needs. This may take the subtle form of a complete hands-off policy, allegedly to offer the child the necessary freedom and chance for self-direction. If this is overdone, it may mean to the youngster: "Mother and father don't love me enough even to care what I do or what happens to me—they never did care anything about me, and this proves it."

Obviously, the possible varieties of neurotic parent-child relationship are too manifold for any attempt at comprehensive discussion here and the foregoing patterns are merely illustrative.

Parents of adolescents face a corresponding task of interpersonal readjustment. Just as the adolescent must revise his image of himself in relation to others, especially his parents, so parents need to revise their picture of him and their role in the relation, as mother, father, and child evolve a changed new basis of attachment. Successful realignment is easier, like all changes, if accomplished over a long period rather than abruptly attempted. This same principle of gradual accommodation has been stressed by many as helpful to the smoother course of adolescent change. Ruth Benedict has shown how certain cultures provide greater continuity and steady, gradual emerging through the stages of development, thus avoiding some of the characteristic disturbances in our society. For parents, too, the ravages of sudden violent rupture can be reduced by emotional preparation.

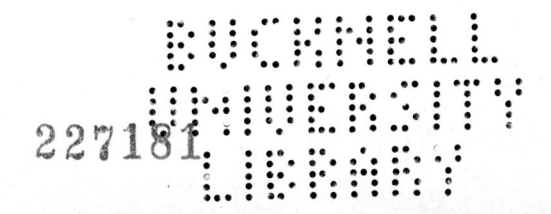

All these parental reactions, added to the inevitable difficulties of growing up, may imperil the success of the task for the youngster. Conversely, the child's adulthood may so shift the parental equilibrium as to precipitate disturbances ranging from the mild and transient to the severe and deeply rooted. The type of impact will vary mainly in terms of the parent's emotional maturity, degree of marital harmony, and healthy nature of the parent-child relation prior to the advent of adolescence.

Often the parents need help of some sort at this time, both for their own sakes and for the indirect value to the adolescent. Family casework is particularly equipped for meeting this need through its understanding of the dynamics of family life and techniques in helpfully applying this understanding. Gordon Hamilton refers to this, saying, "While everyone knows that adolescents need help about their parents, it is not so often realized that the parents of adolescents can be made very insecure by their behavior and also need help." [7]

Caroline Zachry, in discussing general principles of psychotherapy with adolescents emphasizes that for "successfully treating adolescents it is necessary . . . to deal skillfully with the adolescent's parents who almost inevitably present a specialized problem." [8]

Parents who most comfortably survive the problems of their adolescent offspring are probably endowed with a happy combination of tact, humor, understanding, and a gift for emotional acrobatics whereby they can fly through the air with the greatest of ease in response to the lightning shifts between the childish and the adult positions of their young. Such parental psychic agility and forbearance are rewarded by the enjoyment of young people, whose enthusiasms, responsiveness, insistent idealism, and appealing tragicomic intensity can vitalize any household that can contain them.

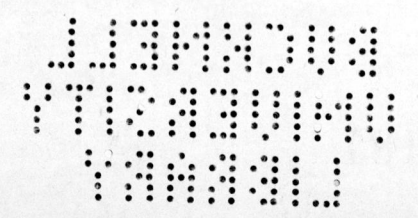

[7] Hamilton, *op. cit.*, p. 285.
[8] Caroline B. Zachry, "A New Tool in Psychotherapy with Adolescents," in *Modern Trends in Child Psychiatry*, ed. Lewis and Pacella (New York: International Universities Press, 1945), p. 80.

Roots of Hostility and Prejudice

ERNST KRIS

THERE HAS BEEN, in the last hundred years, a time lag between the natural and the social sciences, between our expertness in the control of the physical world and our comparative inexperience in the control of social affairs. Awareness of this time lag tends naturally to increase during a transitional period, when the development of the physical sciences has made available energies of great destructive power which cannot as yet be set to equally astounding productive uses. During such a period of transition one may be more inclined than ever to expect from the social sciences counsel on methods that might be used in order to reduce hostile tensions in human affairs, international and intranational.

Speaking from the viewpoint of one of the sciences that owes its importance largely to its position in the borderland between natural and social sciences and has a part in the development of both—speaking from the viewpoint of psychology, so far as it is based on Freud's heritage—I can only confirm that the time lag exists, that we are not equipped as scientists to answer the questions that as citizens seem most important to us. All I can attempt, therefore, is to clarify the nature of some of our hypotheses and the direction in which an increase of our understanding might be expected through coördinated research. Research of the kind we may find most useful will have to avoid the larger issues. It will have to concentrate on areas where systematic observation and, finally, experimental validation are more easily achieved. We have to turn from the areas of international or intranational problems to those which concern the individual's position in his immediate environment, to interpersonal conflict in its various manifestations. We will have to include one further step and center our research on the tensions that arise within the individual himself in consequence of, and as a response to, interpersonal conflict; one may designate this area as that of intrapersonal conflict. It is the domain in which psychoanalytic observation has proven to be most suggestive.

The danger which the hostile proclivities of the individual constitute for any type of social organization has been known to man since the earliest days of self-reflection. Wherever the image of an ideal social order was drawn, from the golden age of myth to the model societies of Sir Thomas More and Edward Bellamy, the absence of hostile tensions became a hallmark of the brave new world. It seems, one is justified in saying, though I do not know that it has been said in so many words, that the absence of aggressive proclivities constitutes utopia.[1]

When we, as readers, follow the writers of utopias into any one of their model societies, we are likely to experience a typical disappointment. After a brief period of interest and after our curiosity has been satisfied, we find ourselves on the threshold of boredom. All is well in the lands of Sir Thomas More and Edward Bellamy. But, in a sense, all is too well. We are likely to resent the sacrifice of individual freedom imposed by the perfectionist planners. Perhaps it is true, as has recently been suggested, that Sir Thomas More did not invent the social order of his utopia; we are told that he based his vision on accounts—peculiarly detailed and understanding accounts, one would have to assume—of Inca society;[2] of a state in which freedom from want was fully achieved, but at the price of total lack of freedom. In this society overt intergroup hostility was minimized, but so was spontaneous resistance against attack from the outside; hence conquerors had an easy time once they had conquered the ruler.

This naturally is not intended as criticism of planning in social life, as implying that social planning and freedom are irreconcilable. The opposite seems to be true. Only planning can guaran-

[1] For a survey see Lewis Mumford, *History of Utopia* (New York: 1923); K. Mannheim, *Ideology and Utopia* (Chicago: 1938).

[2] A. E. Morgan, *Nowhere Is Somewhere* (Chapel Hill, University of North Carolina Press, 1946).

tee and preserve individual freedom, but we need to be aware of the kind of problem we have to face in planning.[3]

Any planning, sound and utopian, starts from the experience that social or institutional change produces changes in the behavior of the members of society. We have come recently to a better understanding of the dynamics of this interaction. While our assumptions are tentative, they open up new vistas. For my present purpose I shall describe these assumptions as consisting of two steps: we are first concerned with the socio-economic situation that requires social and institutional change, and with the individuals who execute it; and, on a second level of investigation, to which we will be able to refer only after a considerable detour, we are concerned with the long-range consequences of such change.

Any specific setup linked to a specific set of social values is likely to attract certain personality types in various functional positions.[4] These personality types influence, in turn, the institutional setup, and modify it through their individual proclivities; hence one may, in fact, speak of the study of institutions as "frozen psychology." [5]

When, after the first World War, the breakdown of the middle class in Germany led German heavy industry and the general staff to the idea of using a new type of mass demagogy to bring about the militarization of German society, this particular function attracted a special kind of mass leadership, rabble-rousers and cranks, most of whom under conditions of a stable social order had failed to make a success of their lives. Our information on the type of National Socialist leadership seems to indicate a high incidence of mental pathology in general and of psychopathic traits in particular. It naturally cannot be assumed that these traits were responsible for the success of the National Socialists in Germany, but I believe that they were responsible for

[3] See K. Mannheim, *Man and Society in an Age of Reconstruction*, tr. Edward Shils (New York: Harcourt, Brace, 1940); L. W. Doob, *The Plans of Man* (New Haven: Yale University Press, 1940).

[4] Heinz Hartmann, "Psychoanalysis and Sociology," in *Psychoanalysis Today*, ed. S. Lorand (New York: International Universities Press, 1944).

[5] A. Kardiner, *The Individual and His Society* (New York: Columbia University Press, 1939).

certain features of the National Socialist party organization, such as, for instance, its specific relation to the submission-dominance continuum and to the part cruelty played in social control. This party organization was, in turn, likely to attract as members and subleaders individuals in whom minimized resistance in submission to authority was combined with a maximized facility in the practice of violence directed against others. One might in these terms describe the most general characteristics of the typical Stormtrooper. Were more detailed data available, we could elaborate on this crude example and demonstrate the interactions between social organizations and types of personality in various areas.[6] For the present purpose it seems more essential that the principle become clear. It rests on three distinctions: we start from a given socio-economic situation, proceed to the institutional setup that (according to the decision of policy-makers) meets this situation, and, finally, to the types of personality that are attracted by this organization. These personalities, in turn, influence the institutions they control and the socio-economic situation that the institutions were intended to meet.

Let me cite a somewhat better documented example: in modern Western society caste barriers and race barriers are no longer strictly institutionalized: Negroes are no longer slaves, Jews no longer live in ghettos. Instead of the older institutionalized barriers that once protected ingroup integrity, that is, the closer allegiance of those who share common interests and common symbols of identification, social prejudice has gained considerable importance: it protects the ingroup against economic and sexual competition by the guarantee of social distance.[7] Prejudice against minorities consequently tends to increase when the level of indulgence of a group is lowered. When life becomes more difficult, for one reason or another, the weaker must yield.

Some authors seem inclined to make the hostile impulses of individuals responsible for the existence of prejudice. This seems

[6] Hartmann, *op. cit.*, has shown that it extends into the field of choice of symptomatology in neuroses and into many other areas of problems.

[7] See John Dollard, "Hostility and Fear in Social Life," *Social Forces*, XVII (1938), 15 ff.; Ernst Kris, "Notes on the Psychology of Prejudice," *English Journal*, XXXV (June, 1946), 304 ff.

a short cut likely to lead to misunderstandings. However, it seems correct to say that the existence of prejudice offers to large numbers of individuals an opportunity of relieving their personal conflicts by offering a target for their hostile impulses. Pressure groups of various kinds clear the ground and make this target more visible; in keeping it before the eyes of the masses they hope to deflect aggressive impulses from other outlets. There are those who, in the service of these instigators, act as agitators. Some case studies concerning American "shirtist" leaders indicate that they are likely to be individuals of various degrees of psychological unbalance. Maladjustments in their personal lives and failures in their economic careers are so frequent as to be almost regularly recurrent factors. They are people with intensely ambivalent attitudes who tend to polarize values. In speaking readily of "the best" and "the worst" they drive their audience from love to hate. Agitators thus strive for the applause which they cannot obtain otherwise, they dramatize their own beliefs and have an uncanny ability of winning others to their viewpoint. With some, this ability serves, subjectively speaking, a particularly important function: they must convince an audience in order to convince themselves.

More detailed and more concrete than these impressions are the data on the personality structure of potential members of prejudiced groups. The investigations of Ackerman and Jahoda,[8] based on data supplied by psychoanalytic psychiatrists, and especially the data collected by Brunswik, Levinson, and Sanford,[9] indicate beyond any possible doubt that, given certain socioeconomic conditions, definite personality features can be established as recurrent in strongly prejudiced individuals. To abbreviate a rather extensive set of data, let me say that we are faced with individuals who in solving their personal conflicts show a high preference for the use of one mechanism of defense: projection. Many of them tend to show marked paranoid features, while others are closer to the obsessional-compulsive type of neurosis

[8] N. Ackerman and M. Jahoda, "The Dynamic Basis of Antisemitic Attitudes," *Psychoanalytic Quarterly*, XVII (1948), 240 ff.
[9] E. Frenkel-Brunswik, D. J. Levinson, and R. N. Sanford, "The Antidemocratic Personality," in *Readings in Social Psychology* (New York, 1947), pp. 531 ff.

than to any other clinical syndrome. In dealing with their scapegoat these individuals follow a universal pattern. The stereotypes that they rely upon are composed of the true characteristics of a relevant number of individuals of the abused group, of characteristics that only a few of its members exhibit, and of general derogatory characteristics that are likely to fit the "typical" evildoer. Scapegoats, briefly, tend to be satanized: in other words, impulses disapproved in ourselves but present in us become the attributes of the scapegoat.

The fact that prejudice functions as a channel of aggressive impulses acts both as a retarding element in the attempt to reduce its social scope and as an impediment to reform. There will be many to defend prejudice, since its tenets fulfill deep-seated needs.

The data on the personality types of extremists in prejudice will, I presume, be supplemented in due course by data on the personality types that are attracted by other social attitudes. Basing our conclusions on clinical impressions we might well anticipate one of the findings that might more clearly emerge: Extremists of all descriptions are likely to show structures that will resemble each other mainly so far as the economy of aggression [10] is concerned. Overt behavior may vary considerably, but the tendency to discharge aggressive energies, against self or others, is likely to play a considerable part. Extremists will then appear as those who are more prone than others to utilize social attitudes for the acting out of personal conflicts.[11]

At this point we turn from the social aspects to those that concern the individual. The question before us is how far our insight into the nature of aggressive impulses in general, incomplete as it is at the present time, can contribute to any investigation of the relation between social change and manifestations of hostility.

Two general assumptions as to the nature of aggressive impulses are usually contrasted; both are derived from the work of Freud, who emphasized both at different times and in different theoretical contexts. According to the older of these views, ag-

---

[10] Cf. E. Glover, *War, Sadism and Pacifism; Further Essays* (London: Allen & Unwin, 1947).   [11] Hartmann, *op. cit.*

gressive impulses (defined here, in agreement with recent writers, as impulses intended to damage an organism or its substitute) arise in reaction to other experiences; according to the second assumption, human beings are equipped with an independent, aggressive drive.

The first view gained wide acceptance through the extensive studies made on the relation of frustration to aggression.[12] Two implementations that have not always clearly been stated seem essential in order fully to appreciate the significance of these investigations. First, aggression is not the only response to frustrating experiences. Secondly, our clinical impressions, supported by some experimental findings, indicate the high frequency with which both insecurity and anxiety stimulate aggressive behavior. It is therefore essential to define "frustrating experiences" so widely that they will include experiences provoking insecurity or anxiety in general. Once frustration in this sense has mobilized aggressive impulses, the first and the second set of assumptions concerning the nature of aggressive impulses need no longer be differentiated for many types of investigation.

The reasons that favor the assumption of an independent drive of aggressive nature cannot be discussed here. They rest largely on the clinical data that only psychoanalytic observation provides; these data seem to many observers to be more meaningful if Freud's latter assumption is applied. What is true of the assumption concerning aggressive drives is equally true of the assumption concerning another kind of drive which Freud designates as "libidinous." Constructs such as these cannot in themselves be verified or falsified, they can only be proven to be useful or useless. They are useful when, based on these constructs, verifiable predictions can be made that could not otherwise be made; in addition, their usefulness is borne out by the part they play in the formalizing of a general theory with which the scientists work.

I assume for present purposes that both these conditions, by and large, have been met and I proceed, therefore, briefly to mention

[12] J. Dollard and associates, *Frustration and Aggression* (New Haven: Yale University Press, 1939); Neal E. Miller and associates, "The Frustration-Aggression Hypothesis," *Psychological Review*, XLVIII (July, 1941), 337 ff.

a further assumption of Freud's: neither libidinous nor aggressive impulses tend to manifest themselves isolated from each other; the degree of their fusion constitutes essential characteristics of all normal and much pathological human behavior, while diffusion of impulses constitutes special types of particularly severe pathology. This assumption is the reason why it seems to be inadvisable to speak, as several authors do, of "constructive aggression."

The libidinous and aggressive drives in the human being are considered as motor powers; but they are considered as sharply differentiated from instincts that in the life of the animal "mediate its adjustment to the reality in which it lives." The properties of the instincts "determine the possible adjustment; with man adjustment is mainly entrusted to learning mediated by independent organization" to the ego.[13] For the purpose of the following considerations I should like briefly to state that we assume that the ego develops out of an undifferentiated structure, that its development is predicated on two developmental series: on the maturation of the apparatus that supplies the equipment for the functions of the ego, that is, for motility, perception, and thought; and, secondly, on the formation of identifications with the early love-objects.

This simplified sketch of psychoanalytic assumptions is inserted here in order to introduce two points: (1) Whenever we speak of the earliest development in the child, of the earliest stages of his ego development, we implicitly describe steps in the tolerance of frustration. Any increase in tension that is not immediately relieved is initially experienced as frustration; hence we may say that frustration is unavoidable and a regular concomitant of any human development. (2) The nature of the human drives, their difference from instincts as known from our study of the lower animals, and the position of frustration in human development account for the role that conflict plays in human life.

[13] Heinz Hartmann, Ernst Kris, and Rudolph Loewenstein, "Comments on the Formation of Psychic Structure," in *The Psychoanalytic Study of the Child* (New York: International Universities Press, 1946), II, 11-38.

Let me quote the words with which a modern biologist and heir to a glorious biological tradition recently formulated this problem. "Man is inevitably and alone among all organisms," says Julian Huxley, "subject to mental conflict as a normal factor in his life and . . . the existence of this conflict is the necessary basis or ground on which conscience, the moral sense and our systems of ethics develop." [14]

With these considerations in mind we are, I feel, better equipped to discuss the kind of data that we would need for a somewhat more detailed study of man's economy of aggression. In studying the present behavior and past history of any individual we will be interested to learn as much as we can about the distribution of frustrations and gratifications in the past and at the present time. But we require, not general, but specific information, especially where the development of infancy and childhood is concerned. We are interested in the distribution of frustration and gratification concerning each of the child's demands, or, to choose a term, in the patterns of indulgence and deprivation to which the individual was exposed.

The data with which we usually operate do not fulfill this requirement. We tend to speak, for instance, of a rejecting or an indulgent mother, but we do not state which of the child's demands were indulged, and which remained frustrated.

A mother may have been highly indulgent to all the needs of the child at the oral stage of his development. She might even have shown a deep understanding of the increased need for her presence that is typical of the second year of life when the child insists on the mother's presence to protect the newly acquired object relationship, resents any kind of separation (here, it seems, is one of the roots of the difficulties of "going to bed"), and reacts to it with anxiety and aggressiveness. But her attitude may be failing when, in the course of his development, the child's interest turns to excreta or to dirt. Then the mother's tolerance may suddenly be replaced by punitive measures. Such sudden shifts and inconsistencies in the mother's attitude are well known so far as

[14] J. H. Huxley in T. H. and J. H. Huxley, *Touchstone for Ethics, 1893–1943* (New York: Harper, 1947), p. 4.

the behavior of the little boy during the initial stages or the phallic phase is concerned, when the mother may react violently to his exhibitionism or his demands for physical proximity. Somewhat rarer are the cases in which the mother's interest is centered on this stage of the development, which she has unconsciously tried to accelerate; such a "seduced" child would, in the framework here suggested, represent but another instance of an indulgence and deprivation pattern. These patterns may be influenced by the problems of an individual mother, but they surely reflect, to some extent, social factors. In a recent publication Anna Freud has drawn attention to the fact that the attitudes of his environment toward the child's libidinous and aggressive impulses can be differentiated according to the class structure. In the lower middle class, oral gratifications are granted comparatively freely, while anal and sexual aggressive attitudes are severely restricted; in the upper middle class, aggression is the main punishable crime, while sexual curiosity is treated more leniently.[15] (These are data concerning conditions in England, they do not equally apply to conditions in this country.)

A young Englishman with upper-class background and progressive leanings was on a government mission and stationed in New York with his wife. A student of Anglo-American affairs, he was devoted to the idea of a mutual understanding. I witnessed the occasion when this attitude was most severely shaken. His young wife had given birth to a boy, and the proud father appeared at the hospital to take his family home. The head nurse praised the newborn heir: "He is a fine fellow," she said. "I am sure he will become a gang leader and beat up the other boys on the block." My friend reacted to this friendly prophecy with some apprehension. The idea that a well-wisher should have wished his son to become a master in externalized aggression instead of in its control seemed to him a peculiarly bad omen.

It would be tempting to generalize from this example and to enter into a discussion of typical British and American behavior patterns, as they seem to be related to the patterns of indulgence

[15] Anna Freud, "Emotional and Instinctive Development," in *Child Health and Development,* ed. R. W. B. Ellis (London, 1947).

and deprivation to which infant and child are exposed in both societies. Problems of this order are, in fact, being discussed under the heading of "culture and personality," or "national character," and a wealth of data produced by cultural anthropologists contains great promise. As yet it seems impossible to isolate any such patterns definitely or to predict their potential influence on formation of character. Too many variables are still unknown. We have spoken of patterns of indulgence and deprivation but in fact we have dealt only with the chronological sequence of both, and not with a number of other aspects in relation to the child's ego development, with the intensity or rhythm with which they were applied, the compensatory devices used, and other factors that in a systematic study of this area will have to be included—data the relevance of which clinical reports usually consider, while in theoretical presentation they are hardly ever mentioned.

These data naturally cannot be restricted, as they frequently are, to earliest childhood. It seems to me that we tend sometimes to underrate the degree to which the character traits and dispositions of children can be molded and modified by later experiences. The progress in our insight is also impeded by the fact that wherever data have been collected, they are viewed more readily in the light of the child's demands for love than in the light of his propensity for aggression. And yet, however closely libidinous and aggressive proclivities are linked in one act, the problems of the individual's economy of aggression are, it seems, to a considerable degree more complex than those of his strivings for love. Let me illustrate this with reference to one of the typical dilemmas. The earliest relationship of the child to his mother is already overshadowed by his ambivalence. When the child, in response to any frustration, experiences hostile impulses—to which the small child is prone to attribute magic effectiveness—these impulses endanger his relationship to, and, in his mind, the existence of, the person that is paramount in his world. While in the preverbal stage of the child's development these fantasies—expressed in oral or anal terms—can only dimly be retraced in psychoanalytic reconstruction, and much in their position and impact is bound to remain controversial, the conflict itself lives on in the child. It reaches its peak during the phallic phase when in both sexes impulses of a hostile nature are directed against rivals who are at the same time the most important love-objects in the child's experience. Under normal conditions in our civilization the father is never only the rival of the little boy, he is also the most important protector from external danger. By the same token the permanent attachment of the girl to her mother is, as it were, only interrupted by the desire to eliminate and to replace her.

These examples are given in order to demonstrate that aggressive impulses are bound to remain incomplete; hence the importance of their fusion with libidinous impulses and the importance of substitute goals and the process of sublimation; hence in education the importance of opportunities for discharge of aggressive impulses in various degrees of competitive and constructive activities. Competitive activities, we may say, are characterized by the fact that at one point a limit is set to the display of violence; that the agreed code of law or fairness inhibits the completion of the aggressive act. In constructive activities the endeavor to solve the problem may be experienced as a battle with an obstacle, as striving for mastery; the structure of the problem to be solved functions here as a limiting factor.

Sublimation of aggressive energy not only leads to its discharge in competitive and constructive activities, in the play of the child and in the work of the adult, but also to another set of processes which we describe as "internalizations." Internalized aggression makes its regular contribution to the formation of the superego and supplies the motor power of conscience. It also manifests itself in a number of other ways, which are as yet incompletely known.

In the formation of the superego the individual's dependence on cultural values can most clearly be traced. Internalized aggression supplies the motor power, but the culture supplies the values for which we stand. I here return to our starting point, the relation of changing social values and human behavior. Effects mediated by the development of conscience do not produce rapid changes. Culture reaches the child through the family, through his parents, whom the child tends to idealize. But the parents, in turn, are not only reacting to a supposedly changed environment, but they carry in themselves values transmitted by their parents —and thus we enter into the chain of traditions.

The nature of the development of the superego in the individual led Freud once to estimate that some of the most important effects of social change would not influence individual behavior before approximately three generations had succeeded each other. I know of no better estimate and of no more exact data to supplement or replace this impression. But it is these data which we need. In order to become meaningful they cannot be limited to one phase of the child's development, to one aspect of his development, and they must be studied with representative samples of clearly defined subcultures. Research of this kind could, I believe, in many ways be advanced by the interest of social agencies.

While exact data are lacking, our clinical impressions lead us several steps further. We know from a study of pathology how far, for instance, the internalization of aggressive impulses can transform human behavior. We know of cultures in which an extraordinary control of the body has superseded the impulse to activity in the external world: it has rightly been said, for instance, that in the practices of yoga autoplastic activity, to use a term of Freud's, has replaced alloplastic activity.

In Freud's thought the idea played a considerable part that the evolution of mankind showed a trend in which the internalization of aggressive impulses was progressing: he spoke in this connection of organic repression, a process that in the life of the species was to be responsible for the decisive changes. Only a part of those hypotheses is subject to empirical validation. But years before the results of current researches in psychosomatic medicine were available, Freud anticipated these findings in stating that the internalization of aggression was responsible for many somatic symptoms.[16]

Freud's thought on organic repression, on changes in the spe-

[16] Sigmund Freud, "Outline of Psychoanalysis," *International Journal of Psychoanalysis*, XXI (January, 1940), 27–84.

cies man, reminds us of the visions that writers of utopias have developed. Their planned societies seem indeed peopled by human beings of a strangely artificial type. Only rarely have these writers explicitly recognized that the internalization of aggression in their societies is bound to affect all the strivings of the individual; that is, that a close link exists in the manifestation of libidinous and aggressive impulses.

When Swift's Gulliver reaches his utopia, the land of the Houyhnhnms, he there finds beings whose life is exclusively controlled by reason. The pains of anger and the tortures of ambivalence are unknown to them. They are not destructive, like the ape men, the Yahoos, of Swift's depiction. But under the control of reason their libidinous impulses have suffered a significant restriction. They cohabit only twice in a lifetime, to procreate the two foals assigned to each horse-couple. They have achieved a lofty detachment from passion, they have preserved individual freedom, but they have sacrificed vitality.

Alternatives of this kind, however vaguely they are anticipated by the intuition of great thinkers, parallel closely some of the questions with which clinicians in psychiatry or education are faced. And yet, extreme alternatives have the tendency to lead thinking astray. Let me conclude, therefore, with a brief statement on what I believe to be recent psychoanalytic findings on useful procedures in handling frustrations of the child's impulses.[17]

In discussing the nature of human impulses I mentioned that they did not in themselves guarantee reasonable gratifications; that the psychic structure of the individual serves the function of mediating between needs and reality. The findings of which I speak seem to indicate that in imposing frustration the growth of this organization can be systematically utilized, or, to put it more generally, that the tension between frustration and the child's needs should be moderated up to a point where frustration becomes self-imposed. The current attempts to reduce the

[17] The interpretation I here present is based on impressions and reports of many workers—of Anna Freud, for one—but I have no right to assume that Miss Freud or any of the researchers whose data I freely use would agree with my interpretations.

Roots of Hostility and Prejudice

earliest tensions by the self-regulation of the feeding schedule of the infant, to postpone toilet-training to the time when the muscular equipment will be adequate, are the best known examples of a tendency in which the growth of the ego apparatuses is utilized. The attempts to use the child's insight, his understanding so far as possible in other areas, the attempt to postpone especially the restrictions of his aggressive impulses, not only until firm object relations exist—until love, for example, is firmly established —but also until substitute activities can be adopted, would be another. In each of these areas and in many related ones in which systematic study has recently been started unambiguous results may not emerge in the immediate future. The complexity of the problems is such that only years of coöperative endeavor and the studies of life histories of children raised under variant but somewhat controlled conditions may permit us to disprove, confirm, or qualify the expectations based on the clinical impressions of psychoanalysis, that the experience of the ego in the control of drives may have a lasting influence on future personality development and hence on man's economy of aggression.

I started to inquire into the relation of social change to the economy of aggression. I conclude by speaking of procedures and techniques that might possibly serve the same end, and yet they have grown out of the initial stages of our research. In fact, one might claim that with every step we take in the advance of psychology as a science, we become less dependent on social values. And yet let us not overlook the fact that even such an attitude is rooted in definite cultural predispositions. If we succeed in the attempt to transfer the rearing of children from the areas of education, with its dependence on the philosophies of life, into the area of mental health, with its dependencies on principles of biology, this will presuppose the existence of a certain set of social values, a certain openness to social change, briefly, what one used to call a "good society."

Part II: Health and the Family

Child Health in Relation to the Family

MARTHA ELIOT, M.D., *and NEOTA LARSON*

MAN SEEMS IMPELLED TO GO ON generation after generation and century after century seeking power, raising issues, precipitating disagreements that periodically lead him to make war on his neighbors. To live at peace with ourselves, with our neighbors, and with the larger community of nations, appears at times to be an ideal that is unattainable. Yet none of us wants to think that this is so.

To seek the answer to such vast problems through the discussion of such an everyday subject as child health and its relation to the family and the community may seem a very small approach to a gigantic world problem. Many wise people, however, have believed in its possibilities. Many students believe that one of the most fundamental things we can do about world problems is to enlarge our concepts of child health and to broaden our methods of attaining it.

This is both a new and an old idea. While Milton could write in *Paradise Regained* that "The childhood shows the man as morning shows the day," he and his generation did not know enough about cause-and-effect relationships to determine the factors in childhood which would make for a healthy maturity. We still do not know enough, but we know much more than Milton did and more than we have found ways of becoming responsible for.

It has been the task of the United States Children's Bureau since 1912 to center public attention on all aspects of child life, to keep the public aware of the fundamental issues involved in the neglect of childhood, and the importance to the total life of the nation of providing appropriately for the child's physical and mental health and his welfare. The Bureau has long been concerned that the family should have security enough—economic, social, and emotional—and knowledge enough to assure that the years of the child's growth and development are years of sound physical and mental health.

The International Health Conference held in New York City in July, 1946, drew up a constitution for the World Health Organization. This constitution sets up certain principles which are basic to the happiness, harmonious relations, and security of all people. One of these principles reads: "Healthy development of the child is of basic importance; the ability to live harmoniously in a changing total environment is essential to such development." The framers of this constitution were thinking beyond satisfactory physical growth when they used the words "healthy development." They had in mind a degree of physical, mental, and social well-being which would assure a generation of individuals so mature emotionally that they would be able to live at peace with themselves, in harmony with the group with which they lived and with all kinds of people all over the world. The greatest task lying ahead of us is to see that we lay a firm foundation for such healthy development of our children, and open the way for steady progress toward its achievement.

We have a considerable body of knowledge about the prevention of certain communicable and nutritional deficiency diseases, the environmental protection of the child from disease and accident, and the protection of the child through the care of the mother during the maternity and lactation periods. During recent decades there has been a rapid accumulation of knowledge with respect to the emotional development of the child.

We have learned much about how to put our knowledge to work effectively in the realm of physical growth and health, but we have not applied this universally, nor have we learned how to persuade society that it should be done. We have lagged even farther behind in the realm of mental and emotional health, partly because of the incompleteness of our knowledge of human psychology and the influence of cultural patterns, partly because of our lack of understanding of how to communicate ideas to each other, partly because we know too little about how people incorporate new ideas into their living and being. We have come to realize, however, how important the family setting is for a child's health, and how important the community setting is for the family's health.

It is obvious to everyone that the health of the infant at birth is directly determined by the health of his mother, by his inheritance from his mother and his father, and by what happened to him during the prenatal period. It is obvious too that the infant cannot exist by himself. If, for some reason, his own family cannot or does not provide him with the care he needs, society must make some provision for him.

Through the preschool years, the years of school age, and during the transition from adolescence into adulthood, the child lives, not "in relation to the family," but as an interacting part of the family. In a very fundamental way, the family shapes the destiny of the child. Just as fundamentally, each child by his very presence in the family, by his characteristics, by what he wants and gets from the family, and by what he gives to it shapes the destiny of the whole family. There is no more important quest for knowledge than that of finding out more about what these family relationships mean, how they affect the way in which a child lives and grows, and how they affect the kind of a human being he is and becomes.

If the child is to be healthy, he needs a life which is satisfying to him at whatever age he may be. He is not merely a future citizen. When, as a newborn infant, he is first cuddled and nursed and held closely by his mother, his sense of security is strengthened, his fears are allayed. He at once becomes a member of the family. He belongs. Everything that happens to him or his family from this time on affects his future mental health for good or for ill. When we discuss child health, we are talking about something that grows as the child grows, something that cannot be postponed. We cannot ignore the urgency of the period of childhood for every child.

The child's physical health cannot be separated from his mental health. Physicians and research workers in the fields of psychology and psychosomatic medicine have amply demonstrated this. The child who is frustrated within his own family, who is not sufficiently loved, or who is too rigidly controlled, may become insecure in his own life. He may thereby be unprepared to deal emotionally with a physical illness that in a secure, stable person would be minor and passing. He may unconsciously be seeking illness as a way out of his insecurity.

We cannot ignore the fact that it is much easier to concentrate on a problem of sickness than to face the problems of the normal growth and development of the child. It is natural for our sympathies to be enlisted by a visible handicap. There is drama in centering our attention on it—pain in our failure or our inability to provide the child the help he needs. We must have eyes to see also the deeply moving drama that unfolds as we assure the optimum conditions of growth and development for all children.

There is excitement and happiness in a normal pregnancy, a strong baby carried to full term, a mother and father loving each other and their newborn child. There is satisfaction and pleasure in looking forward to giving the care and affection needed to meet the demands of the child's physical and emotional development. It would be unusual, however, if parents did not at the same time have feelings of uncertainty in relation to this new experience, if they did not sometimes have feelings of anxiety about how they were going to measure up to their new responsibilities. A mother and father will frequently need the help of doctors, nurses, nutritionists, social workers, who understand the normal emotional problems of pregnancy as well as its physical aspects.

There is an excitement and pleasure that come to the father and mother as they watch the baby grow and develop week by week into a normal, healthy toddler, and then as they see him become more and more of an individual, month by month, year by year. The baby's health and well-being is positive and dramatic fact to his parents, particularly in his early years.

Child Health in Relation to the Family

A periodic appraisal of the child's development by a doctor specially trained in pediatrics, and the discussion of his findings with the parents, is important at this time. As the child grows and has a greater physical independence and is able to do more things for himself, the parents begin to express need for help in handling behavior situations which may be a normal part of development but which they may not be prepared to understand.

This periodic appraisal of the child's growth, this availability of professional help for use when parents need it, is what we are seeking. All too often—and this is true for doctors as well as for social workers—interest in the child who is developing normally flags. It is easier to wait until he becomes sick, or presents a behavior problem which is so severe that his parents are helpless in the situation, before giving him our specific attention.

It is right that we treat children who are physically and emotionally sick—there is no question about this—but we must go deeper into the problem. We must forestall illness. We must build health. We must place a continuously greater emphasis upon health—health interpreted as the most favorable growth and development of the child. Care which is provided for children when they are sick is included in this concept, a concept geared to the total health needs of the child and not merely to a sickness which he may have. The foundation for this kind of medical practice now exists in modern pediatrics.

Educational programs are needed more than ever before to inform parents what good child health is, what we mean by positive mental health, what the relationship is between physical and mental health, and how to work toward good health as the objective for their own children. Doctors, nurses, social workers—all the personnel with professional responsibility for children—must be much better trained than they are now in the knowledge of the normal child, so that they can give this kind of help to parents.

How practical are these ideas? How far can we expect them to reach out to the children of this country?

If this kind of health and medical service is to be of use to the individual child, it must exist within reach of where he lives. The basic preventive services that are given in well-child clinics, in doctors' offices, in community services for school children, must be accessible. The headquarters of the public health nurse must be so conveniently located that she can get to any child's home as often as she is needed. Social services must be within reach.

Many doctors are not now trained to care for children in this way. Ways and means must be found to bring to the general practitioner the newer concepts of child health as well as to increase the number of doctors who specialize in care of children. The services of specialists must be made available as needed, through a state and local plan which will either bring them into the locality where the child lives, or which will provide for taking the child and his parents to the services.

It may not be possible to have a fully equipped diagnostic service and hospital located in every neighborhood or community. In many areas there are too few people to justify establishing and maintaining such services. Where this is true, practical arrangements must be made to give emergency care locally and to provide transportation to the nearest hospital or clinic.

This is roughly the statement of a standard. Let us glance at what exists in the far reaches of our nation—the today out of which tomorrow will develop.

Many children live in areas where the ratio of physicians to population is unfavorable. Other children who live in states where this ratio is favorable are deprived of the kind of health and medical care they need because the doctors are either too busy to give them the time and attention that they should have or are unequipped to do so. In approximately one third of the counties in the United States there are no public health nurses to serve families and children. Almost three fourths of our rural counties have no regularly established child-health clinics.

In many areas of our country, there are not enough hospital beds. For the most part, outside the big cities, sick children are hospitalized in the adult wards and often go without the special pediatric care which they ought to have. In many parts of the country, facilities for the care of Negro children are not so good as those for white children. Care for children in families of mi-

Child Health in Relation to the Family

grant workers is usually inadequate. In relatively few communities are there pediatricians or general practitioners who have been trained to approach the child and his parents with a positive and constructive plan of mental as well as physical health service.

We know that for large numbers of our children, health and medical services do not exist within reach of the place where they live. There is not enough trained personnel. We need more doctors, dentists, nurses, nutritionists, social workers. Many of the professional people concerned with the health and well-being of children need an opportunity to keep up to date on the newer methods of child care. There is difficulty in getting highly trained people to settle in some of the more thinly populated areas which need service.

This is one part of the problem. If the services were freely available, could families with children afford them? To safeguard the health of the mother and her child both before and after birth, the family must be able to afford adequate food, housing, clothing, and other essentials of life, as well as health and medical care. We would like to believe that the American standard of living assures these essentials to all families, but when we look at the statistics, particularly as they relate to children, we find that this is not the case.

Children are concentrated in low-income families. Slightly more than half of our children live in families whose total family income is $3,000 or less. Two thirds of them live in families with total family incomes of $3,500 or less.

Children are also concentrated in the low-income states. The 1940 census showed that about one fourth (28 percent) of our children live in the Northeast, which has 40 percent of the national income, while another one fourth live in the Southeast, which has only 12 percent of the national income. There is no reason to believe that these ratios have changed materially since 1940.

Rural areas are particularly at a disadvantage. Many are impoverished. Farm families have the highest ratio of children to adults, approximately twice that of the large cities. In 1941, for instance, farm families had 29 percent of the children in the United States and only 11 percent of the income. Their purchasing power in terms of health and medical care is necessarily low.

It is obvious that many families with children cannot afford medical care, or, when they do afford it, it is at the expense of other essential items. Even comparatively rich families find themselves wondering, indeed worrying, about whether they can afford the health and medical care they need when an expensive illness strikes. Often a family whose income is between $5,000 and $10,000 finds it difficult or even impossible to meet the cost of care for a child suffering from cerebral palsy or rheumatic fever, or from other conditions which are costly to treat.

Obviously, we are not talking merely about the relatively few people who come to social agencies for financial help, or even the larger group who are receiving public assistance grants which by medical standards would, in almost all parts of the country, be inadequate to assure the kind of health care that we want for children. We are talking about the many persons who are, in general, self-supporting but who cannot meet the costs of maternity care and child rearing at the standard required for positive health.

We see no answer to this dilemma except by finding some way of pooling funds to meet all the costs for care of the child in health as well as in sickness. In my opinion, this can be effectively accomplished only through public programs, where all the people contribute on the basis of their ability to pay and where public responsibility assures that the services and facilities required to meet all the needs of the child in the family will be available.

There are those who believe that voluntary prepayment systems will solve the problem. This seems unlikely, particularly for families with children, unless government makes the payments into the system in behalf of a large number of families. This is an uneconomical way for the people to provide care and one that is likely to introduce the "means test" into its administration.

Whatever the method, it is evident that we should not have two systems of health and medical care—one for those who by some standard are judged to be able to pay for such care out of their own resources, and another for those who are not able to do so. We believe heartily in the objective of health and medical care available to all children in the same way as education is today. As Grace Abbott, second chief of the Children's Bureau, said many years ago: "The sources of revenue must be as broad as the causes of need." Some of us may live to see the day when this principle has been accepted as a measure of the public responsibility that all people bear for the health of our children.

As we examine the problem in this way, it becomes obvious that there is a planning job which has to be done for the child in his family—one which involves the family but in its scope is beyond the responsibility or ability of the individual doctor or the single family to solve. If known standards are to be met, if we are to make available to the child in the family the skills and knowledge which we have, the community, the county, the state, and the nation must assume an increasing responsibility. The families that make up the community must unite in a concerted effort to develop the kinds of resource which are needed for the physical and mental health of their children.

This does not mean that the family can, or should, give up its individual responsibility for the child. The role of the community, in the broadest sense of that term, is to make the family's job possible and truly productive in rearing children who, to quote again from the constitution of the World Health Organization, have the "ability to live harmoniously in a changing total environment."

We have already spoken of the meaning of this job of rearing healthy children to the future peace of the world. It is not only what nations do for their children that will count, it is how well the individuals who make up nations, especially parents, learn through a variety of ways, applicable to their own culture, to understand the elements of child care. It is how well they understand and can be responsible for the influence that their own life experiences may have on the way their children's mental development takes place and emotional maturity is reached.

We have an ever increasing understanding of the emotional life of man, an ever increasing understanding of why children grow to maturity with behavior patterns that result in individual and group conflict and prevent "harmonious living." A vicious circle exists. Parents who do not understand themselves or their own attitudes and conflicts bring up children who reach maturity and, in turn, become parents with the same attitudes and conflicts. To learn how to break this vicious circle, we need more research in the basic and applied social sciences, as well as in the biological sciences. We need also to discover how to make the knowledge we have more effective in the lives of individuals, in family relationships and in larger groups.

In 1950 there will, no doubt, be a fifth White House Conference on Children. This mid-century conference will be able to look back at a record of fifty years of unprecedented increase in knowledge and skills in the physical care of children. Stock will be taken of the great advances in controlling communicable and nutritional diseases, of the amazing declines in the infant and maternal death rates. The country will be able to congratulate itself on the progress made in the assimilation of the new knowledge of how to protect the physical growth and development of children in the routine practices of family and community life. Furthermore, there will be reports on the advances that have been made during recent years in understanding child behavior and the bearing that the parent-child relationship has on the emotional development of children.

The Conference, however, if it undertakes to evaluate honestly the present status of our achievement, will recognize that an unknown but probably large number of children have reached maturity healthy and strong in body, but insecure and unstable in their emotional development; they have become adults unable to live in harmony with themselves or others, unwittingly translating their own inadequacies into aggressive behavior and into belief in the necessity of war between neighbors and nations as a method of solving disagreements. Indeed, the Conference will have to face resolutely the fact that unless the situation is changed, one out of every twenty children alive today will sooner or later find himself or herself a patient in a mental hospital.

This mid-century conference will, we believe, turn its atten-

Child Health in Relation to the Family

tion quickly and deliberately to the great job that lies ahead. The second half of the twentieth century should be devoted with steadily increasing effort to the development of a new preventive mental health service as part of the regular child health service, one in which families will participate, and through which the fundamental practices of good parent-child relationships will become as much a part of the everyday activity of families in rearing children as are the rudiments of infant feeding and the control of smallpox and diphtheria today. The turn of the half century might then mean the beginning of action that will result in a generation of mature youth, well adjusted to life in our democracy and as world citizens, able to live at peace with themselves, with their neighbors, and with all kinds of people all over the world.

In such a movement the family will hold the center of the stage because it is into the family that the child is born; it is in the family that he will first learn to control his feelings of jealousy, fear, aggression, or inadequacy; it is in the family that he will first learn to understand the rights of others; it is in the family that he will learn to be so confident and secure in his relationships with others that he will have no need to be either too aggressive or too repressed when he moves out as a more independent social being into his life at school and in the community.

Though the family will hold the center of the stage, it will need the support of the community and the nation. To find the way to build a generation of young people physically and emotionally mature, healthy and strong, able to meet successfully the task of living together in relationships of mutual trust and confidence, able, in turn, to raise still another generation of cooperative human beings, is our most important job. This is no idle or impractical dream. It can be done if we direct all our attention to it. It may seem visionary, but "where there is no vision the people perish."

Pioneering in London: the Peckham Experiment

INNES H. PEARSE, M.D.

THE PECKHAM EXPERIMENT, with its laboratory, the Pioneer Health Center in London, is an experiment in the field of human biology. It is an attempt to study the power or "urge" behind human living, as any physical scientist might set out to study any form of energy in the physical world. The experiment presumes the existence of such an energy or "urge." It also presumes that its evolution will be found to follow certain natural laws, and that those laws will be ascertainable. It presumes, lastly, that where human beings can align themselves with natural law we should see an ordered pattern arise in society as well as a great enhancement in living itself within that society.

From the outset we are faced with immense experimental difficulties; for, while in the physical world the physical scientists are dealing with uniformities of equal or equivalent quantity, in the living world we are dealing with total diversity: no two identical fingerprints the world over; no two similar individuals in any society we might choose for observation. From the outset in this experiment we leave the measurable realm of quantity and enter the, as yet, unmeasurable field of quality. It is probably difficult to appreciate the significance of this without an understanding of the spontaneous nature of health.

A good deal is known of how order is sustained in the plant and animal world and something of the ecological balance between organism and environment in both these fields. Hitherto, the experimental scientist has not turned his attention to the nature and circumstances of order in the great and unexplored field of human biology, that is to say, in human society. Whenever a sustained pattern has arisen it has been of spontaneous occurrence and has resulted from instinctive action rather than from a knowledge of natural law.

On the other hand, we have a vast knowledge of disorder, physical, psychological, and social, in man and his society. Strange to say, it is commonly assumed that this knowledge of disorder, by some inverse equation, gives us an equal and valid knowledge of the nature of the order. Who is the expert on health?—the doctor. Who is the specialist in psychology?—the psychopathologist. Who is our chosen adviser, in social planning?—the economist and the social worker. Yet in Great Britain the social worker is there by reason of the social ills that have to be assuaged—sickness, poverty, delinquency, break up of marriage, etc., all of which demand an immediacy of action which is first therapeutic and then preventive rather than cultural in its operation. By "culture" I mean "growing," not the variety of culture often spelt *Kultur,* nor even "culture" as it is understood by the educationist.

The medical profession, which assumes the major responsibility for health, is in a similar situation. Its informative science is that of pathology, the science of disease and disorder. Pathology has progressed through the study of susceptibility to disease. In the phenomenal strides that have been made in this subject we have as yet failed to ask the all important question; not, how disease spreads, but how it is that some persons escape it. For example, in every epidemic there are those who, although exposed, do not "take" the infection or do not succumb to the disorder. What, then, is the nature of their insusceptibility? We know much of the circumstances that cause the reaction of disease. We have yet to study the conditions that engender an actional relationship of ordered ease between organism and environment. We know much of sickness and its processes; we know nothing of the processes of health. What is health: and how is it sustained? It was to find an answer to this question that the Peckham Experiment was devised.

The first requisite for such an experiment was to select healthy specimens of society for observation and to secure circumstances in which such folk would come voluntarily within the field of experiment. Peckham was chosen as an area within our metropolis in which we were likely to find the most healthy specimens of society—neither too rich, nor too poor, intelligent enough to hold down good jobs, independent and competent enough to paddle their own canoes without help or direction. Its people were no social problem group or underprivileged people but a fair section through a wide range of class, wage, and culture. Voluntary association in continuity between this group and those conducting the experiment was achieved by forming a health club available daily for the leisure of its members.

The second step was to gain some idea of the physique of each individual who joined the club. This determined one of the very few conditions of membership in the club—a periodic health examination for all who joined. What we, as biologists, attempted to do was to make a *health* examination, that is, a search for what is right. This is to be distinguished from a *medical* examination, which is a search for what is wrong with the individual.

The result of this procedure has been to give us information as to the degree of diagnosable disorder in those who believe themselves in "health." That is a very interesting disclosure,[1] but not one that is necessarily pertinent to our own studies. Much more pertinent is the fact that in the small number, roughly 10 percent, of those found to be without diagnosable disorder we do not necessarily find the vitality and capacity for action—for living—that one would anticipate in health. These were often people who were only half alive, people unaware of the significance of their surroundings, too diffident to explore them—undeveloped people.

Our experiment has told us that the absence of disorder is no measure of health. Health is not, in fact, a static entity; it is processional, in organism and in environment. Health lies in an actional relationship of organism and environment, both evolving in mutual synthesis. In health, organism and environment are

[1] George Scott Williamson and Innes H. Pearse, *Biologists in Search of Material* (London: Faber & Faber, 1938). Innes H. Pearse and Lucy H. Crocker, *The Peckham Experiment* (London: Allen & Unwin, 1943; New Haven: Yale University Press, 1946).

The Peckham Experiment

inseparable; they are mutually related, one living by the other. So the meaning of health is something nearer to the old intuitive meaning of the word "wholeness." Its synonym is holiness, that is, relatedness within a greater whole.

That being so, we must cease to use the words "health" and "sickness"—whether in relation to cure or prevention—as interchangeable terms, as is the current usage. In Britain we assemble, in one building, clinics for the early detection and treatment of tuberculosis and venereal disease, for the extraction of tonsils, for infant welfare and antenatal care, we add to it a mortuary for the housing of the dead pending burial, and we call the institution a health center! We do not even blush for the writer when we read in the morning paper that a new chair of child health is to be inaugurated, the object of which is "to deal comprehensively with all the diseases of childhood." I believe that the same confusion of language obtains also in the United States, for I saw recently the health activities of a community center billed as lectures on tuberculosis and venereal disease!

It is a strange and new field into which ethology, that branch of human biology which is concerned with the study of natural "order" and ease in man, is leading. The new field of investigation has demanded new material and new instruments. Instead of operation theaters, dispensaries, and glass cages to isolate the newborn infant from its new-found environment, the new types of instruments required are opportunities for action, such things as swimming pools, theaters, playgrounds, musical instruments, dance floors, cafeterias—all of them environmental media that are conducive to personal and social action in a fluid and free environment.

The Pioneer Health Center—pioneer because it set out on this quest—is, in fact, a "laboratory" equipped with just such instruments for the continuous use, in their leisure, of those living in its vicinity. The features of its building are large, open floor spaces, interrupted only by supporting pillars, so that there are no enclosed rooms or cul-de-sacs limiting free circulation. As well as free circulation everywhere there is also everywhere free visibility. This is secured by glass partitions wherever an enclosed space is essential, such as the chamber of the swimming pool, the gymnasium, the theater. The nature of the building, constituting an open forum in which there is free circulation and free visibility for all at all times, is an essential condition of the experiment; for we set out to find out what people would do when they could do what they liked, when they liked, where they liked, and with whom they liked.

Now as to the nature of the material under observation in this laboratory: with what biological "unit" were we to work? We had set ourselves the task of investigating the natural order of growth and development in a specimen of human society. In the great process of evolution we had discerned two phases held in equilibrium. One is that of "senescence," demonstrated by the individual who can only grow older and older; the other, that of "juvenescence," by which novelty and diversity are introduced into living. This process of juvenescence is manifested only by the mated pair. Neither male nor female alone could thus demonstrate to us the full scope of human growth and development. It is through having children that the individual comes to full maturity, that the male becomes a man, the female a woman. And it is through the child that the new is born into society and society is diversified. It is not, then, with any "unit," as in physical science, but with a functional "unity" that we had to deal in setting up our experiment. That caused us to define as "family" this unity of the mated pair which holds the biological potentiality of children within an intimate, biologically specific environment—the home. So a mother and father with several children and a young married couple without them are equally "families" in our sense. In either stage of growth they represent a unity with the potentialities for juvenescence or the anewal of society, as well as for senescence or individual maturation. Clearly, we could not use the individual as our unit. We had to work with the family as our "unity." This is not merely a practical desideratum; it is a biological concept of fundamental importance.

So our laboratory is peopled with families. No individual can join without his family. Hence the subscription for membership is a family one, the same whether for a young couple just married or for a mother and father with any number of children. Before the war it was one shilling per week per family; since the war and at the express desire of the families, it has been increased to two shillings per week per family. This sum is low enough not to exclude from membership a family with a low wage.

What does this family membership mean in equipping the club? There must be equipment affording opportunity for action for people of all ages, for the infant, the "under fives," the school child, the adolescent, as well as for parents, whether young or old. Still more important in a building planned for free circulation everywhere, it means that all ages mix and mingle throughout the club, just as people do at home.

I understand from what I have heard and read of American life that in the United States such a situation would he highly unusual. I gather that there is a great gulf between the activities of parents and those of their adolescent children. Let me tell you what happened in our experiment. For the first ten months, parents, with their infants and their school children, used the Center freely. The adolescents could be seen putting their heads around the door: "Mum and Dad's there: come on—let's get out of this." Apart from their attendance at their health examination—a condition of family membership—they were seldom seen. Only as the membership grew to 500 and 600 families and the grown-ups —particularly the young married folk—began to do things did it become a desirable place to the adolescent. Now, when he puts his head around the door: "Come on, it's all right, Mum and Dad's playing whist." From that time they came in numbers which represented their statistical proportion in society. They were shy and they were awkward or boisterous in their social incoördination. But they were within sight of, and in contact with, that very desirable "big fellow." Result: they wanted to emulate the big fellow and spontaneously began to modify their actions; and in doing so, they had unconsciously moved into the next stage of maturity.

This process of being naturally drawn to further maturity through continual contact with the slightly more mature appears to have general validity in society. Just as the young adolescent wants to be like the older adolescent, so the older adolescent is subtly affected by those couples who are in the serious courting stage; the courting couple grow interested in the newly married. Perhaps the most marked example of the effect of contact with the more mature was to be seen in the young married folk. When they joined it was often with the announcement that they wished to have no children, or no more children. Within two and a half years this desire has been reversed. They now often shyly announce that they want to have a child, or another child. It is important to note that there has been no increase in their wages, no improvement in their inadequate housing accommodation. What released the natural urge to a further maturity? The sight of other families enjoying having children; the enviable sight of other families widening their field of social excursion in the process, penetrating further into and understanding more fully their environment in the course of the natural growth of the family. Health, like disease, is infectious, given the conditions in which its infectivity can operate.

There were in the Center special circumstances which made this a possibility. Interested as we are in growth and development, we keep in closest contact with the family throughout each important phase of parenthood as it occurs. So when the wife becomes pregnant, she is re-examined, and during the whole period of pregnancy the greatest attention is given to nutrition [2] and to the maintenance of all the bodily reserves, as well as to their mobilization through her continued, if not enhanced, activity during pregnancy. This seems natural to the family, for in consultations occurring at each significant stage in parenthood the husband and wife come to regard pregnancy as a natural process —one of ease, not of disease—and one through which they, as parents, can reach out to their own full maturity. So, since both of them are assured that everything is in order, are assured of the great capacity of the latent reserves now being called into action, the wife confidently and with zest continues all her activities and

---

[2] In order to secure food of known quality and freshness the Center has a farm as an integral part of its equipment, the produce of which is primarily used for families in which there is pregnancy and for the children in that family who are under five years of age.

interests. She swims, she plays badminton. Indeed, to their surprise, both parents find that through this very pregnancy they are being led further and deeper into their social environment. They meet others who also are about to have, or have just had, a baby, and out of common interests, friendships grow. Now this is possible only because of the family orientation of the Center, and because of the possibility for continuity in its many-sided, day-to-day contacts. Here mothers may meet while making layettes or with their children in the afternoon; in the evenings, the husbands come in, and the families mingle. Where at a parental consultation courage may have seemed lacking and understanding not complete, either or both may be engendered by the actions, the understanding, and the experience of other families. Gossip and seeing what others do are fruitful methods of infection with these qualities of courage and understanding. The Center is a place where gossip tends to lose its idle character and becomes a vector of topical education. Knowledge spread in this way has the advantage of being transmitted in the vernacular. It becomes part of the idiom of the people. It reaches them at the time when their "ears are open" and when they can forthwith use it. This is an example of what we have defined as "topical family education."

So the pregnancy proceeds. Two days before delivery the wife is swimming in the pool, two hours before she goes to the hospital she is in the cafeteria with her friends; forty-eight hours later she is back at home with her baby, visited daily by the Center midwife. There is the minimum dissociation from husband and home. She gets up directly she is ready to do so and attends to her own child. The parents bring the baby as soon as possible to the Center for his first examination, and for a further parental consultation. Here they find out all they can of how the baby is growing, and come to recognize the meaning of the new orientation his presence is bringing about within their family circle. So they carry on till the time of weaning approaches, the time for the next parental consultation.

So greatly and so quickly did the families appreciate these services that by the end of two and a half years in the Center we had young people coming to ask if they could have their next health examination advanced so that they could be as fit as possible by the date of their summer holiday when they hoped to "start a baby." We had with quite unexpected rapidity reached the hygienist's dream of parents voluntarily seeking to free themselves from disorder before conception occurs.

In the Center we go further. I have said that only families are eligible as members. To that rule there is one exception. The grown-up son or daughter of a member family is allowed to introduce a boy or girl friend as a temporary member. The temporary members have full use of the social activities in the Center though they do not have the privilege of periodic health examination. In this way the young people acquire a far fuller range of opportunity than they would otherwise have of doing things together and with others, within the setting of a mixed society of all ages during the years that they are moving slowly toward the discretionary choice of a mate. When a final choice is made and marriage is in view, each then has the privilege of examination followed by a joint premarital consultation. So we have moved toward the eugenist's dream also, of easy, diverse, and graded contacts for selection of a mate, within a mixed society, with knowledge of the significance of marriage as marriage is approached, and the full advantage of medical science to diagnose and to eliminate disorders before wedding.

All this sounds perhaps a little facile. Why, if it is apparently so easy, do we not see the unfolding of living energy more frequently in our own families, in our friends, and in our social organizations? One of the features of living organisms is the possibility of arrested growth. If circumstances are not favorable, existence continues, but growth and development are not manifested. The circumstances for full growth and development have not been present in ordinary life in our metropolis.

What, then, were the circumstances peculiar to the Peckham Experiment? I have already mentioned several of these: first, the family orientation of the club with its corollary of a society consisting of all ages mixing freely in their associations and in the use of all material; secondly, the periodic health examination by means of which all eradicable disorder is removable at the outset; thirdly, the easy contact between biologist and members, so that the family is able to take such information as it can make use of at the time when it is ready to embody it in its daily life and actions. As one member said, "I've been thinking, Doctor—we've got a swimming pool downstairs and to enjoy it we've got to learn to swim. Upstairs, we've got a 'pool of knowledge' and, like the swimming pool, to enjoy it we have got to learn to swim in that too."

But there are other salient factors in the Center which allow life to go forward in ease and order rather than in disease and disorder. In the Center there is material for action of every sort, set out in such a way that it and the use of it are visible to all. We postulated that the sight of action would prove to be the natural stimulus to action. This we have found to be the case, but with certain modifications. It is taken for granted by the educator and by the social organizer that the sight of expert achievement is the stimulus to achievement. We find this to be the case for the small number who know what they want to do, and who have some capacity, however small, for doing it—a mere 10 percent or less of the populace. What of the 90 percent of the adult population who do not particularly want to do anything and who have little skill or accomplishment? For them, the natural stimulus is the sight of someone less competent than themselves doing something that they feel they could do as well, or better. The wife of forty who since marriage has foregone all physical activity other than her housework is heard to say to her husband as she sits by the window of the swimming pool, "Jim, look at her! She must be ten years older than me, and with that figure too! I don't see why I shouldn't go swimming." A week later she appears in the swimming pool.

The significant observation to be made here is that it takes contact with all sorts to provide the natural stimulus to action. Had the only swimmers all been experts, the swimmers would form a select and progressively exclusive group, surrounded by a crowd of spectators—as we see on our playing fields and in many of our best equipped community centers. The cult of the expert within the community engenders social aloofness and militates against participation of the people as a whole in social action. Moreover, nonparticipation to any degree at all ultimately means noncritical and invalid spectatorship.

It will readily be seen from what I have said that were the families to be drawn from one class, one wage level, one type of industry, or from one grade of education, the foci of stimulus to be found within the group might well be too limited to evoke anything like full function in the family. In choosing Peckham as our locality, it was this very possibility we had in mind. Peckham was a residential area where there were congregated within a square mile families with a wide diversity of culture, wage, and occupation. We had calculated that 2,000 such families, that is, 10,000 individuals, would give us one or two good musicians, one or two actors, one or two good football players, and so on, who by taking advantage of the material available to them in the Center, would inject their enthusiasm into the families gathered there. Were we to have chosen, for example, a new housing development where there were people of one class, one type of skill, we should have needed a center to accommodate 100,000 individuals in order to insure a diversity of interest within the group. In the absence of such diversity what could be done but to introduce such interests through the services of organizers and leaders? But in doing so we should have dammed back the springs of spontaneity and initiative, foreshortened growth and predetermined social action.

The fact that the families are of varying wage, education, social class, and skill means that there is within sight and knowledge of every family a great diversity of experience. This enables us to dispense with leaders, teachers, experts, and professionals and organizers. In the Center there is none of these; there is only material for the use of all the members. The absence of all instructors, leaders, and organizers is an unusual circumstance obtaining in the Center. Members can do what they like, when they like, how they like, and with whom they like. As they use this material they discover others who want to use it too. That leads to getting together to find how to arrange so that each can have his use of it and all be satisfied. That very necessity leads to an awareness of the "other." A very different inference would be tacitly drawn if an organizer were to step in and formulate a program. Each individual then would be confirmed in the insistence upon his "rights" set against an anonymous "other" or "others." The sense of wholeness would be undone rather than enhanced, and separateness would be perpetuated.

By segregating people into social and economic strata, as we have been doing since the Industrial Revolution, we are quelling the natural flow of living, robbing all classes of the natural stimulus to discretionary action, making impossible the natural "infectivity" of health, destroying the "wholeness" of society. In so doing, it may well prove that, to cope with the absence of these very qualities of vitality and discretionary action in society, we are saddling the future with a burden of health and educational administration that may well prove too heavy to be borne. In social life we are, in fact, doing much the same as we are doing to the sources of human food: first we process out the vital quality, and then we proceed to administer as a drug the "vital" elements in artificial form.

Man does not live by bread alone but by all that he can take from the endless diversity of his environment. If there is insufficient diversity he will suffer a fractional starvation of his personality. He will retire and encyst himself, or he will break out and disrupt the social environment. In either case, the springs of action are quelled and ordered living is inhibited.

But as the social worker only too well knows, every degree of both these reactions exists in society, quenching the flow and disturbing the emergent energy that, suffusing the family, should lead to the fullness of living.

Unlike the sources of physical energy—coal, petroleum, and water power—found in vast deposits, living energy is scattered. It is distributed in small unities—"families." Dispersed throughout the social matrix, it is families that emit biological energy, like nuclei of cells within the body tissue. If something is faulty in the function of each nucleus, if the living energy cannot flow freely from family to family, from home to home, then there can be no cohesion, no strength, and no power in society, no "organization" in the biological sense, however great the systemization, however intense the planning.

The seed of social order is the family. If we wish to "grow" health we must cultivate the soil or environment through which the family must feed to function. This is the first natural law that has grown out of our study of human biology. That, given favorable circumstances, biological "energy" is evolved through the family has been demonstrated beyond question in the Center. We have seen that this energy, given freedom of action as one of the favorable circumstances, will quicken a group of families, leading them to orientate their living on a mutual basis to the advantage of all. In biology the correct term for this is "organize": take shape, form organs which, through growth, become coördinated, by which we mean the manifestation of a spontaneous order in their living.

To a biologist this is no surprising finding, for he knows that there is no "leader" sealed up within the egg to direct the growing chick. Order is immanent in all biological material. But biological material has to wait on circumstance for its urgent unfolding.

Maintenance of Health: Exploring in New York

BAILEY B. BURRITT

As a boy and young man, I loved to read of the doings of explorers. The vivid, fascinating accounts of their experiences, especially those in the north and south polar regions, interested me much more than fiction. Exploration has a universal appeal. It suggests pioneering, bold imagination, careful analysis of the field, planning with precision and discipline, patience, and courage in action.

The maintenance of health is almost as much of a mystery as the still only partially explored Antarctic region. It is a relatively new concept in the field of health and medical care. Our medical libraries have volume upon volume on how to treat people who are sick. The percentage of medical literature dealing with how to keep people well is growing but is still small; and, in my lay judgment, it is in no way commensurate with the scientific knowledge available as a basis for a more extensive and profitable discussion of the subject.

This is, then, an interesting and important theme. It will be recognized at once that any thoughts that I may develop on the subject are those of a person whose experience has been in the field of social work. For many years it was my privilege to be associated with the New York Association for Improving the Condition of the Poor and, later, with the Community Service Society. Over the years I have had abundant opportunity of observing families which have been deprived of the economic, social, and individual satisfactions of life which might have been theirs had more attention been given to the maintenance of their health.

Let us turn our attention to some of the underlying reasons for our exploration. Perhaps the most fundamental of these is that the approach to the problem of the maintenance of health has been predominantly that of locking the stable after the horse has been stolen. In other words, society, through both its medical profession and its social institutions, has devoted its thinking, professional energy, and funds for health purposes primarily to the care of the sick instead of the maintenance of health. An examination of the relative time and attention given to the care of the sick as compared to that devoted to keeping people well in the actual private practice of physicians is convincing evidence of this. A comparison of the amounts expended by any of our leading municipalities and states for health departments and other preventive services as compared with those spent for hospitals, institutions, and organizations caring for chronic and other types of illness is even more convincing.

If we examine the curricula of our medical schools we cannot fail to be impressed by the great amount of time and thought devoted to training in therapeutics as compared with that devoted to the science of keeping people well. While progressive, forward-looking professors have been increasingly including instruction in the preventive aspects of medical science, the relative amount of this in most medical schools is still out of proportion to the need. Significant evidence that the trend toward greater emphasis upon this phase of training is quite recent will be found in the fact that not until the decade of the thirties did most of the five great medical training institutions of Greater New York establish full-time professorships of preventive medicine. The visiting nurses organizations of New York City, in close touch with the problems of families in their homes, have made every effort to direct the attention of the public and of practicing physicians to the importance of doing more preventive educational work with these families. But the care of the sick whose needs are pressing has swallowed the larger part of their financial resources as well as the time and energy of their professional staffs. More adequate financial resources would make more preventive teaching possible.

The nursing staff of the Community Service Society is devoted entirely to health instruction and has done much pioneering work in the prevention of sickness. The Department of Health of the City of New York, devoted exclusively to prevention, is the most extensive factor in providing such services to individual families. Some of the services, such as those that provide a pure water supply, pure milk, etc., affect all the people in the city. Other services, such as those devoted to the protection of the health of mothers and babies, are directed in increasing volume to the prevention of illness in particular families.

It is important to give full credit here to the obstetricians and pediatricians whose practices are primarily concerned with the maintenance of health. These men have rendered great service in pioneering and demonstrating the possibilities of this type of practice, with the result that families have learned that compensation of physicians for keeping patients well is a good investment. This lends credence to the belief that they can be led to see the advantage of applying this principle in other forms of medical service. An increasing number of progressive physicians in fields other than obstetrics and pediatrics are deriving satisfaction from giving their attention to the maintenance of health of their patients, and there is evidence also that an increasing number of thoughtful people are looking to physicians for help in their efforts to keep well and are showing greater willingness to pay for this help.

However, when we bring together all the various preventive services of the city and appraise their extent and significance, we are impressed with the small volume when compared either with their importance or with the extent of the therapeutic services of the city. And even in the existing preventive services there is inadequate instruction of families with regard to the steps that are desirable and necessary to keep people free from disease.

We find, then, that in any fruitful exploration and pioneering in the maintenance of health in New York City we must be concerned with developing ways to direct increasing attention of medical schools, practicing physicians, nursing organizations, public, municipal, state, and Federal officials, as well as of the people themselves, to the importance of learning how to keep well.

May I now point out some of the difficulties which the Community Service Society has experienced in directing its attention to the importance of developing or modifying present health services to place greater emphasis on keeping people well? The work which the Society has done with families over the years has led to recognition of the fact that preventable illness is a very large factor in developing a need for social services and economic assistance. ("Preventable" as used here refers to either the complete prevention of disease or the prevention of serious disability resulting from disease.)

Sickness plays such an important part in the economic and social problems of families that the Society has accepted the general principle that a careful medical and social appraisal of the family and its individual members is necessary as a basis for its program of helping them to help themselves. It has tried repeatedly, but always with indifferent success, to secure from existing community facilities such a sound medical base for its educational and social services as would be afforded by a careful medical examination of all members of the family, or at least of any members apparently not in normal healthy vigor. In those cases where persons are obviously ill, it has been possible at hospitals, or at the best out-patient services of the city, to secure for them both examination and treatment. In cases of those not obviously ill, this attention has not been available, and the Society has been reluctantly compelled to provide a limited and inadequate amount of diagnostic service for these people at its own expense.

This points to a serious lack of services directed to keeping people well. If the Community Service Society, with its good will among hospitals and social service institutions, cannot secure health appraisals of persons who are not obviously sick, certainly individuals with modest means cannot hope to procure such help. Even persons with sufficient means often find it difficult to get the most helpful guidance. This is due, in part, to the fact that both the training and the practice of physicians are centered mainly on treating people who are sick. Many physicians have had little training or experience in advising people who are concerned primarily with keeping themselves free from disease. We preach unceasingly the importance of early diagnosis to prevent the development of uncontrollable illness, yet we practice almost exclusively examination and treatment of people already sick. Too often the sickness is well advanced. How can we keep people well if we give them no medical guidance until they are ill? Are not periodic appraisals of the health of all persons a necessity for progress in the maintenance of health?

Let us now examine an additional reason why exploration of matters affecting the maintenance of health is desirable. The very rapid development of physical and chemical science has made possible great strides in medicine. At the same time, it has made it well-nigh impossible for the medical student to keep abreast of available knowledge and skills that are necessary if he is to deal with the medical needs of his patients with even reasonable competence. This has led to a rapid trend toward specialization, which, while having the advantage of placing greater skill at the disposal of people, also has disadvantages.

One of the disadvantages is the disappearance of the family physician who knew each member of the family, was well acquainted with their relationships to one another and to the community, and was a real friend. Few practicing physicians now have this intimate personal association with families. Another disadvantage is that the extension of the science of medicine has brought great pressure upon the time and energy of the physician to keep pace with the rapid development in the scientific facts underlying his profession. His training and the pressure to keep abreast have caused his attention to be focused more and more upon the developments in research and the laboratory with the result that his patients are too frequently treated as cases rather than as human beings. While the individual has benefited by the increased knowledge and improved techniques and skills placed at his disposal, he has, at the same time, been deprived of the advice and guidance which in the past his physician, having full and intimate understanding of his personality, was able to give him.

The pressure of rapidly developing science upon medical practice also has tended to retard recognition of the fact that each person, in addition to being an individual, is an integral part of a physical and social environment that is constantly influencing his personality. The health of the individual is closely related to the health and social habits of his family. It is as a member of that family that he lives in a home, eats his food, secures his rest, and is continuously exposed to good or bad health conditions. It is here that most of his intimate personal relationships are developed. It would be of considerable significance in the maintenance of health if both physicians and families were to accept the concept that the family is the unit in medical practice. This is particularly true if the maintenance of health is the major objective.

In this examination of some of the underlying reasons for exploration in health maintenance it is possible that we may have discovered some useful clews for further experimentation. We might learn much, for example, from a well-conceived and thoughtfully directed experiment in medical practice which would rest on the foundation of keeping people well with the family as the unit of procedure. Such an experiment, with a limited number of families over a number of years, would give us valuable experience with regard to the advantages and limitations in this approach to the problem. Can families be interested in keeping themselves well? If so, can they be sufficiently interested to pay the cost? What modification of present practice is essential to shift the emphasis at once to the family as the unit with the objective of keeping that unit well? These are some of the questions we might try to answer in such an experiment.

If an experiment were found desirable, might it not include a thorough health appraisal of each member of the family and such observation and reappraisal as experience proves practicable as an essential basic concept? This would involve new procedures and additional expense. Further progress would be made in determining what procedures are effective in keeping people well. There is still considerable uncertainty with regard to this. We would learn whether the expense of caring for the sick might be lessened, and whether the total cost of good medical care is greater or less through such an approach. Would this bring about earlier detection of disease and tend to correct it before it became disabling? Would individuals and families welcome such an approach to the conservation of their health? Would it tend to make them overconscious of the possibility of developing disease and thus have an undesirable effect upon their well-being? Experimentation should help to answer at least some of these questions.

Our preliminary exploration points to the desirability of weaving the concept of health maintenance more closely into the pattern of group practice of medical service. Group practice is increasing rapidly. It is being experimented with in diverse forms in widely scattered geographical areas. In New York City it is still in the age of infancy, learning how to stand and walk alone. Progress here and elsewhere, however, is convincing thoughtful students that this form of medical practice offers distinct possibilities for improving and extending medical service. At present, however, both public and medical thinking about health maintenance has limited experiments in this field primarily to group practice in the care of the sick. What is needed now is an experimental demonstration in group practice in which the main objective is health maintenance. If such an experiment were feasible it would give a fillip to promising progress of group practice in filling the gap created by the gradual disappearance of the family physician.

It is an acknowledged fact that health maintenance and therapeutics are practiced more or less separately, whereas it is now recognized that only through complete integration of these two aspects of medical practice can the best results be obtained. A serious and prolonged experiment to enable us to learn from experience how these services can be most effectively and economically integrated would be both timely and profitable.

Reference has already been made to the present tendency of science and scientific techniques to overshadow the fact that all patients are personalities living and moving in a social setting. Recognition of this in practice is important. Pressure of time makes it difficult for the physician to secure full advantage of this social factor unless his skill is supplemented with that of the trained social worker and public health nurse. An experimental demonstration that undertakes to ascertain under carefully controlled conditions how the skills of these professions can be successfully integrated and focused upon the health maintenance of families in their occupational and social environments should yield fruitful results. This would tend to demonstrate how important the consideration of the personality and social environment of individuals and families is in the effort to keep people well, and how various professional services can be successfully combined in the attainment of this objective.

The medical student of today is the precursor of the medical services of tomorrow. Medical students now are receiving more training in prevention of disease than they did formerly. Nevertheless, their training still lacks emphasis upon health maintenance. A student has but little exposure to the best methods and practice in health inventories of individuals and families. His observations as a student and intern are still made predominantly, if not exclusively, in hospitals and in the care of the sick. Public health would improve more rapidly, and perhaps the total volume of illness might be lessened, if the point of view of medical training could be oriented more definitely with reference to the main objective of keeping people well. In any event, more adequate opportunities to observe the best of preventive services, and more instruction and observation in the science of the best practice in keeping people well, should result in greater well-being and less disease without loss of the best possible care to those who become ill.

Prepayment for medical care is now accepted by the medical profession and the public as a desirable method of distributing the costs of medical care so that persons in need of such care will assuredly be able to procure it when they need it most. There is still considerable difference of opinion as to how prepayment can most efficiently be administered. A variety of experiments is now under way, and from the experience of these we shall learn how we can best resolve these differences. We need now to add the objective of prevention of disease and the maintenance of health to the present objective of using prepayment as a means of bringing prompt medical services to a larger number of sick persons. Only in this way can the full benefit of prepayment be realized. Prepayment for the avoidance of illness is surely as valid as prepayment for the care of sickness.

Does the exploration which we have been attempting point to the next fruitful steps? It has seemed to the Health Maintenance Committee of the Community Service Society that it does. This conclusion grows directly out of the long experience of the Society in dealing with many thousands of families. It is stimulated and confirmed by the experiment which has been so thoughtfully conducted over a period of years by the Pioneer Health Center of the Peckham Experiment in London. The committee has received further inspiration from its review of some of the trends toward health maintenance in the best of American experience. It would like to see a well-controlled experimental demonstration undertaken over a period of years in efforts to learn more definitely from actual experience what advances can be made in the prevention of illness and keeping families well. Such a demonstration should be sponsored by, and directly affiliated with, one of the great medical training schools of the city in order to insure the best standards of care, thoughtful scientific direction and maximum opportunity for instruction and observation of medical students. The committee believes that medical service in such an experiment should be provided by a group practice unit in order that the benefits and difficulties of such practice could be explored more fully. Believing as it does that the family, with the interrelationships of its individual members, is of fundamental importance in medical service, it would make the family the basic unit of this demonstration and would limit the families to such number as could be given adequate, well-planned, and directed care. In full recognition of the fact that keeping people well requires attention to the social environment of the family and also accepting the fact that maintaining health is closely related to thorough and intensive health teaching, the committee feels that these families should have available, not only the various skills of physicians, but also those of the well-trained social worker and public health nurse. This would have the added advantage of affording opportunity to see how these various professional skills can be integrated most successfully and economically.

The selection of families that are already providing for their home as well as for hospital medical care on a regular weekly, monthly, or annual payment basis would perhaps be desirable for the experiment. This would make it possible to experiment with the addition of preventive and health maintenance techniques to the medical care already provided through existing prepayment services for a group of such families as might be interested in more intensive efforts to keep in a state of health. In this way, we would learn what preventive and health maintenance techniques are effective and practical, and how persistent and sustained interest of families in keeping themselves well can be maintained.

We realize that the organization and successful conduct of such an experimental demonstration would be difficult. It would require a careful delineation and definition of objectives. It is perhaps too inclusive as outlined. It might be found that the demonstration as proposed would be endeavoring to find experimental answers to too many unanswered questions. To be successful, such an experiment would have to be conducted over a period of years if results capable of being woven into the general pattern of medical care were to be found. Responsibility for the executive direction of such a project would need to be delegated to a physician with great understanding of human nature as well as a thorough knowledge of medical science. It would be a social as well as a medical experiment.

In any event, in plans for such a demonstration much thought would need to be given to provision for suitable means of measuring results. A selected group of families, similar in make-up and environment, could perhaps be followed up as a control group. However, the fact that this would necessitate keeping two groups of families under continuous observation over a considerable period of years presents difficulties. Whether this particular method of measuring the scientific results is worked out or not, the point I wish to emphasize is that unless great care is given to plans for securing reliable scientific measurement of results, it will not be possible to speak with certainty as to the answers which are being sought to these questions.

Such a program obviously could not be undertaken without provision for meeting its cost over and above the income which might be derived from the families cared for. The Health Maintenance Committee believes that the Board of Trustees of the Community Service Society is prepared to make available over a period of years limited funds for such a program, provided competent direction and leadership in a suitable environmental setting are assured. If this could be done and a pioneering effort of this nature undertaken, it would be the expectation of the Community Service Society that further significant contributions might be made to the health and well-being of our population.

Health and Family Life: Health Maintenance

THOMAS D. DUBLIN, M.D., DR.P.H.

ONE CANNOT OVEREMPHASIZE the far-reaching significance of the Peckham Experiment in London in redirecting needed attention to the meaning of that overworked and yet poorly understood term "health." I must confess that it has not been easy for me to grasp all the implications of the concept of health which has been developed in the Pioneer Health Center, namely, the ability of a family and its component parts to move through life —to grow and to act spontaneously—with ease, with order, with vitality, and with human dignity. Perhaps this is a frank acknowledgment of the effect which the predominant emphasis on pathology in my own medical education has had upon my thought processes. Only relatively recently have I been able to comprehend fully the potentialities of an attempt to determine as a physician what is right with people rather than what is wrong, and to visualize how such information may be utilized in helping people to enjoy fuller, richer lives. That the pioneers in London have given medical educators food for thought is confirmed by the simple question which each person might well ask himself: "How often have I gone to my own personal physician and, after a thorough and careful interview and examination, been apprised of all my assets rather than my defects?" I am willing to gamble that, at best, we have been told: "I can find nothing wrong with you."

Though sociologists have recognized for a long time that the family is the functional unit of our society, it has remained for the Peckham workers to develop a valid concept of family health and to demonstrate all that it implies. It is such patient and careful observations as Dr. Innes Pearse, Dr. George Scott Williamson, and their co-workers have made over a period of twenty years which provide a sound basis for the claims of medicine as a social science. I am reminded of Rudolf Virchow's prediction 100 years ago:

> Should medicine ever fulfill its great needs, it must enter into the larger political and social life of our times, it must indicate the barriers which obstruct the normal completion of the life cycle, and remove them. Should this ever come to pass, medicine, whatever it may then be, will become the common good of all. When we have exact knowledge of the conditions of existence of individuals and of peoples, then only will it be possible for the laws of medicine and philosophy to gain the credence of general laws of humanity.[1]

I feel perfectly justified in saying that the pioneering studies of the Peckham Experiment have been requisite for the explorations of health maintenance in New York. Only with such fundamental observations on which to base our plans has it been possible for groups such as our own to propose a program of health services applicable to conditions existing here. We do not intend to emulate in detail the Peckham program. Rather, we aim to profit by the lessons to be learned from that experiment and to utilize the techniques of health maintenance which have been thoroughly tested there. It is noteworthy also that in England, where the devastation of the recent war has made rebuilding of whole communities necessary, the Peckham idea is being woven into the pattern of community planning. I understand that in Coventry, in Bristol, and in a number of other British cities, the experience gained in the Peckham center, the laboratory, is being translated and applied on a broad social scale. The centers in these cities too will be laboratories, and yet over and above that they are concrete efforts to meet social needs.

It is in this relationship that I see at least one major departure from the basic concepts of Peckham in the plans we are developing in Brooklyn for a program of family health maintenance. Because of the specific focus of the Peckham Experiment, it has been somewhat less concerned with the provision of medical care

[1] Rudolf Virchow, *Die Einheitz bestrebungen in der wissenschaftlichen Medicine* (Berlin: Druck und Verlag von G. Reimer, 1849), p. 48.

required by those departures from health to which we are all subject than with the study of families when they are well. Only 10 percent of the members of the Family Club at Peckham were found to be free of disease or disorder at their initial health examination, and an even smaller fraction were found to have the vitality which health connotes.

In our thinking, we have been unable to escape the conviction that if health or "wholeness" is our goal, we must concern ourselves with all phases of health and medical care for the selected families we hope to include within our demonstration. Thus, in our planning, we hope not only to merge health promotive measures with those of prevention, treatment, and rehabilitation, but, in doing so, to utilize the group practice of physicians and of other necessary professional personnel. In addition, we intend to incorporate the prepayment principle, in order that the cost of services provided may be brought within the means of those families for whom these services have been designed. We envision a new type of family physician who will serve as the key member of this group as well as the coördinator of all services required for healthful living. It is upon this family physician that we shall place immediate responsibility for the guidance and health care of the family, and through him each family and each member will be assured continuity and individualization of service. Perhaps here the true function of the doctor, as teacher, can be achieved.

We are mindful that at Peckham the health examination is considered as quite apart from a medical examination and medical care as now generally conceived. We do not believe, however, that the physician or medicine itself is at fault, and that this is so because medicine has its roots inextricably buried in the science of pathology. We are inclined rather to lay the responsibility upon our present, and in my opinion outmoded, methods of medical education. Though it may be difficult to overcome the inertia within our present medical school curriculum, we are hopeful that the medical training of the future can be built in larger measure upon the science of ethology, the science of health. To do so, we must have, if not a Peckham, something akin to it, where our students may learn about health and not solely about disease. We also visualize that through such a center we can bring into our team of teachers those who have been trained primarily in the social sciences as well as those traditionally trained in the biological ones. To the social worker and the public health nurse I would like to add others, as, for example, the anthropologist and the social psychologist, who, I am convinced, could help us to solve many of the health and medical problems which thus far have escaped solution.

Constructive Medicine and Positive Health

HENRY E. MELENEY, M.D.

ONLY BY READING the little book entitled *The Peckham Experiment*,[1] seeing the pictures of the Pioneer Health Center in operation, and examining in detail the method of operation, can one fully appreciate the vision and detailed planning which went into the experiment, and the happy results which have been obtained. The principle which struck me most forcefully in reading the book by Dr. Innes H. Pearse and Miss Lucy H. Crocker was that a single human being is not a complete biological unit but that biological union of the male and female is necessary to create this unit which is the family. It may sound trite to repeat this principle which is perfectly obvious, but ignorance of it is certainly the cause of one of our great gaps in the medical field. The Peckham Experiment, it has been said, is an experiment in human biology, and is certainly much broader than an experiment in social health as a background for physical and mental health. It has set the social stage for the all-round development of the family and has provided facilities for periodic observation of the physical status of the family in the social setting.

The social progress of a family or of a group of families, such as is being studied by the Peckham Experiment, is, I suppose, a most difficult thing to measure without long observation. The criteria for measuring such progress must be extremely difficult to establish. Undoubtedly, the maintenance and promotion of physical health may be measured as a result of the periodic in-

[1] Innes H. Pearse and Lucy H. Crocker, *The Peckham Experiment* (London: Allen & Unwin, 1943; New Haven: Yale University Press, 1946).

Medicine and Health

ventory, but this is certainly only a part of the picture which may be developed as a result of the broadening of the social outlook through participation in the activities of the Pioneer Health Center. Dr. Pearse expresses a modest satisfaction with the success of the program thus far, but I hope that at some later time she will report what concrete results have been obtained in the maintenance and promotion of the physical health of her families other than the diagnosis of abnormalities and their correction or control. Perhaps we may have a comparison of the incidence of manifest disease, infant death rate, marriage rate, or birth rate in her families with those for the Peckham area as a whole. I know, of course, that in all public health work it is often difficult to show by statistics the value of specific procedures, and particularly of services which are not directed against one simple problem; but it would be of interest to those of us who would like to see this type of experiment conducted in the United States to have such facts in addition to a general appreciation of the philosophy and methods of the Peckham group to use as an argument by which to obtain the necessary facilities for a similar experiment in the United States.

One of the interesting features of the Peckham Experiment is the fact that it seems to be entirely independent of the medical services which must be required from time to time by the member families. I understand that such services have been deliberately omitted because of the basic philosophy that health is the goal of the experiment. On the other hand, there is the theory that there is value in associating the study of well families with a medical institution or medical group which can supply both preventive services and services at the time of illness. It will be interesting to see how we can reconcile these differences in points of view.

It is obvious that a functional building is necessary to put into practice the philosophy of the Peckham Experiment. Moreover, it seems to me that another requirement, which I gather is met in the Peckham area, is a relatively homogeneous population with regard to racial background, religion, customs, and what we ordinarily call "general culture." I wonder whether we could find in New York, with its heterogeneous population groups, an area in which such an experiment would be as successful as it appears to be in London.

The Community Service Society of New York first approached the problem of the family from the social point of view, later developing a medical and educational nursing service when the social importance of health was appreciated. In contrast to the Peckham Experiment, this work has been done with selected families having obvious needs and scattered over a wide area of the city. It has been done by work with the families in their homes rather than in a center and it has grown up on a service basis, for those who already have problems in social pathology, rather than as a deliberately planned experiment in the promotion of health. It has been an extensive service in contrast to an intensive experiment such as the Peckham experiment. Here we might ask whether working in the homes of families has certain advantages which counterbalance to some degree the advantages of observing families in a center. Are people perfectly natural when the social worker or nurse calls at the home? On the other hand, are they perfectly natural when they are observed in a center? Undoubtedly, in either situation a complete understanding of their biology depends upon the degree of confidence which they have in those who are directing, or attempting to direct, their activities.

On the social side, a study which is associated with a medical group, if it were lacking a recreational center, would presumably use the recreational facilities ordinarily existing in the community and would doubtless attempt to improve such facilities wherever possible. The wide variety in quality and attractiveness of such facilities in any area in New York and the lack of any unity in their programs would certainly make it much more difficult to persuade the families to use them effectively. Furthermore, many recreational centers in New York are supported by, and cater to, certain racial or religious groups, which may be advantageous from a practical point of view but cannot attain the goal of encouraging the breakdown of social barriers.

I believe that there may be certain advantages in maintaining and promoting the health of well families in New York in close association with a medical center which has the facilities and aim of maintaining and promoting health as well as of diagnosis and treatment of physical ailments. Such a medical group can furnish premarital advice, antenatal care, obstetrical service, postpartum infant and preschool supervision, immunization, periodic health inventory with the necessary laboratory examinations, and dental care as well as office or home visits for those who are ill, hospitalization, surgical attention, and other specialized services as indicated. Social workers connected with the group can visit the homes of families. Nurses can also visit as health educators as well as for bedside nursing when needed. And the physicians in charge of such a study, who should, of course, be human biologists, could visit homes both when the families are in health and when illness occurs. Such a group, in order to fulfill its highest function, must continually examine its services to be sure that it is giving maximum emphasis to constructive guidance toward positive health. Parenthetically, I may state that New York University, in remodeling its medical curriculum to meet the needs of the future, is planning to change its Department of Anatomy into a Department of Human Biology.

The establishment of a control group for such an experiment in New York would undoubtedly be extremely difficult. If the member families for a control group were enrolled in a prepayment plan for health and medical services they would thus at the outset be a selected group, and the very fact of their being observed, without receiving direct health promotion services by the staff of the study, might influence their health and social activities. If they were not enrolled in the prepayment plan, they would probably not be comparable to the study group in many ways.

Personally, I feel that the Peckham Experiment is so epochal in its conception and development that it should be repeated in some form in the United States; perhaps an inland city where the population is more homogeneous in racial and religious background would be more suitable than New York. Wherever such an experiment is established, I believe it would be most advantageous to construct a recreational center and to place it in close proximity to a medical center and a public health center. Incidentally, I should like to emphasize that in our public health centers we have health promotion activities such as well-baby clinics and school health supervision in addition to clinics for the diagnosis and treatment of certain diseases. I am confident that financial support for a Peckham Experiment in the United States could be obtained and that personnel with the vision and social outlook of the Peckham group could be found who, after a first-hand study of the Peckham Experiment, could adapt it to American conditions.

I should like to call attention to the increasing eagerness of people in the United States to make use of opportunities for a periodic health inventory. One illustration of this is the growing popularity of health maintenance and cancer-detection clinics which are being established in many cities. Adults are willing to pay a reasonable fee for such inventories. Already, the clinic established in 1947 at New York University has made appointments six months in advance. True, its clients are individuals and not families, and they are mainly people who think that they may have some physical defect or who have had cases of cancer in their families. However, in industry also there is an increasing provision and demand, not only for preplacement examinations, but for periodic health inventories, and both management and labor are beginning to appreciate the economic and perhaps the social value of such service.

Finally, I wish to call attention to a study in China which may at first not seem to be relevant but which I believe has within it certain qualities which are similar to the philosophy of the Peckham Experiment. I refer to the Mass Education Movement in China, founded and promoted by James Yen. It was established in a rural community in North China for the purpose of decreasing illiteracy. In developing the project it was found that four elements were necessary: first, education, in order that the people could read and write; secondly, improvement in agriculture, so that the people could take advantage of their literacy by becoming economically self-supporting; thirdly, the improvement of

Medicine and Health

health; and fourthly, the institution of honest local government. This movement has been such a success that it is now being started on a province-wide basis in Szechwan Province in West China. Since therapeutic medicine in China cannot be developed for centuries as it has been in the Western world, the country must emphasize the maintenance and promotion of health and the prevention of disease. China thus has the advantage of us in standing on its own feet and building from the ground up, and it is time that we stopped standing on our heads in emphasizing curative medicine more than preventive and constructive medicine.

The Next Generation—Its Nutrition and Health

BERTHA S. BURKE

THE POSSIBILITIES for improving the health of future generations involve many factors, and reliance cannot be placed upon any one approach. To obtain maximum results, attention must necessarily be devoted to the protection and promotion of the health of every individual at all stages of life from conception—even prior to conception—to full maturity and thereafter. At all stages of life we must use every known means for the promotion of physical fitness, resistance to disease, and mental and emotional well-being.

Dr. Thomas Parran has said that "tomorrow's civilization can be made vastly different and far better than today's, if we put to work now, what we know now about the nutrition of human beings." [1] So also Professor Henry C. Sherman, of Columbia University, has said: "Our newer knowledge of the relations of food to health is one of the major advances of modern science, and perhaps it is outstandingly the one on which each of us can act everyday for the life-long well-being and happiness of ourselves and our children." [2] In the years which lie ahead, as the science of nutrition is better understood, it will assume an increasingly important place in our public health programs and in other aspects of preventive medicine. Again quoting Dr. Sherman, it is "through wise daily living, and notably through intelligent food habits" that it is possible to provide "such a favorable

[1] T. Parran, "The Job Ahead," in *Proceedings of the National Nutrition Conference for Defense* (Washington, D.C.: United States Government Printing Office, 1942), p. 219.
[2] H. C. Sherman, *Food and Health* (New York: Macmillan, 1947), p. 3.

Nutrition and Health

internal environment of body as shall permit our inherited abilities to develop and function to the best advantage."[3]

One of the parent organizations of the Community Service Society, the Association for Improving the Condition of the Poor, realizing the importance of nutrition in relation to family health, was the first social agency to appoint a nutritionist to its staff. This position, created in 1906, was held by Winifred Gibbs, who was especially interested in food and food economics as related to health.[4] In 1913 three more nutritionists were added to the staff, and in 1917 the organization established its Nutrition Bureau under the able leadership of Lucy Gillett. Through this service over the years the Community Service Society has been a forceful pioneer in translating into simple everyday ways of living for its clients the research findings which would lead to better growth and development of infants and children and improved health of the family. This interest in nutrition as it may affect the family continues. It is to organizations such as this that we must continue to turn for the practical interpretation of the results of research to the communities which they serve. Their breadth of vision and their ability to interpret scientific knowledge in terms of everyday living will help to shorten the interval between scientific nutrition findings and the application of this knowledge to the nation's families.

As a nutritionist who has become deeply interested in the protection of the health of the child-bearing woman and her offspring, through attention to the adequate satisfaction of nutritional needs, I shall devote my attention first to nutritional problems as they may affect pregnancy. This period, particularly in regard to nutrition, has been and still is the one most neglected in the life of the child. Therefore, well-planned efforts further to improve prenatal care would seem to be the logical starting point in an attempt to improve the growth, development, and health of future generations. It has become apparent from studies of human beings as well as animals that environmental factors operat-

[3] *Ibid.*
[4] *Report of the Subcommittee on Nutrition: Nutrition Service in the Field.* White House Conference on Child Health and Protection (New York: Century, 1932), pp. 60–64.

ing through the mother may affect the course of embryonic development and fetal growth and thus modify the outcome of genetic potentialities. Changes in temperature, and in the chemical composition of the environment which may be the result of nutritional inadequacy, may profoundly alter embryonic development in animals. Furthermore, there is evidence that certain diseases occurring in the human mother at the critical stage of embryonic development may alter seriously its course. German measles is a striking example which has become recognized in recent years.

In devoting my attention to the evidence as to possible nutritional factors which affect the state of well-being of the infant at birth, I am not overlooking the possibilities of many other advances which may contribute toward a far larger percentage of infants being wellborn. I hope to show that nutrition is one important environmental factor which deserves consideration in all prenatal care programs. In future planning for the improvement of child health much more consideration must be given to the growth, development, and health of the fetus. The life of the individual begins with conception, not with birth, and between these two events much transpires of profound importance for the future well-being of the individual.

Normal physiological processes of the body are greatly altered during pregnancy. Digestion and absorption from the intestinal tract are frequently impaired, especially during the early months, and nutritional requirements are considerably increased during the latter part of pregnancy. Pregnancy is, therefore, a period of stress and one during which evidences of nutritional deficiency are likely to appear. Many women in this country enter pregnancy in a poor nutritional state because of poor food habits of long standing, which are the result of ignorance, lack of money, poor appetite, faddism, and the like. It is little wonder, therefore, that the increased adjustments and requirements of pregnancy may result in nutritional failure of varying degrees. In addition to these well-known facts, considerable evidence has been accumulated which indicates that the fetus no longer can be considered a true parasite, and that faulty nutrition may affect, in fact, not only the pregnant woman, but also her fetus in ways that are not usually considered to be the results of malnutrition.

I should like to discuss briefly some of the prenatal studies which have appeared in the literature since 1940. These studies have been carried out on relatively large numbers of pregnant women and have demonstrated a significant relationship between maternal diet on the one hand and the course of pregnancy and the condition of the newborn infant on the other. Several of these studies have included evaluation of the usual diets of the women during pregnancy; in others, known supplements were fed to the expectant mothers, while in certain countries, rationing of food has afforded an unusual opportunity of studying the effects of diet during pregnancy upon both mother and fetus. One of the early studies which has commanded considerable attention is that of Ebbs, Tisdall, and Scott,[5] carried out in Toronto, Canada. Three groups of women were studied during the last half of pregnancy. The diets of the women in one group who had poor incomes were supplemented with food to an excellent nutritional level; the members of another group of women, whose incomes were considered adequate, were taught an excellent diet for pregnancy; while the women in the third group remained on their usual poor diets and so served as controls. The incidence of abortions, premature births, stillbirths, and neonatal deaths was significantly higher in the group on the poor diets. The women in the group with supplemented diets and those who had been taught how to improve their diets not only had healthier babies, but they themselves proved to be better obstetrical risks. These women suffered from fewer complications, including less toxemia, and they had fewer difficulties during labor, delivery, and the postpartum period. The ability of the mother to nurse her infant also appeared to be influenced by the quality of her diet during pregnancy.[6]

[5] J. H. Ebbs, F. F. Tisdall, and W. A. Scott, "The Influence of Prenatal Diet on the Mother and Child," *Journal of Nutrition*, XXII (1941), 515–26. See also *Milbank Memorial Fund Quarterly*, XX (1942), 35–46.

[6] J. H. Ebbs and H. Kelly, "The Relation of Maternal Diet to Breast Feeding," *Archives of the Diseases of Childhood*, XVII (December, 1942), 212–16.

The People's League of Health of England [7] investigated the result of giving supplementary minerals and vitamins during pregnancy to approximately 50 percent of a group of 5,000 women; the remainder served as controls. The incidence of prematurity was significantly reduced in those who received the supplemented diet. This finding is important, since in England about 50 percent of the deaths of infants under one month of age are due to prematurity. Another English study reported by Balfour [8] included nearly 20,000 pregnant women chosen from the lowest income groups in England and Wales. The diets of 12,000 of these women were supplemented with vitamins and minerals as well as with milk; the remaining 8,000 served as controls. Significant reductions in the stillbirth and neonatal mortality rates occurred in the supplemented group, and the maternal deaths were extremely few.

The Department of Maternal and Child Health of the Harvard School of Public Health, working in conjunction with the Boston Lying-in Hospital,[9] has studied 216 pregnant women drawn from the prenatal clinics of that hospital. Detailed dietary histories were obtained at intervals from these women. An over-all relationship was found to exist between a good or excellent diet during pregnancy and good physical condition of the infant at birth. This relationship is shown in Figure I.

Ninety-four percent of the infants born to women whose diets were good or excellent were in good or excellent physical condition at birth. In contrast, 67 percent of the infants born to

[7] "Interim Report of the People's League of Health: Nutrition of Expectant and Nursing Mothers," *Lancet*, II (July 4, 1942), 10–12.
The People's League of Health, "The Nutrition of Expectant and Nursing Mothers in Relation to Maternal and Infant Mortality and Morbidity," *Journal of Obstetrics and Gynaecology of the British Empire*, LIII (December, 1946), 498–509.

[8] M. I. Balfour, "Supplementary Feeding in Pregnancy," *Lancet*, I (February 12, 1944), 208–11.

[9] B. S. Burke, V. A. Beal, S. B. Kirkwood, and H. C. Stuart, "Nutrition Studies during Pregnancy: I. Problem, Methods of Study and Group Studied; II. Relation of Prenatal Nutrition to Condition of Infant at Birth and during First Two Weeks of Life; III. Relation of Prenatal Nutrition to Pregnancy, Labor, Delivery and the Postpartum Period," *American Journal of Obstetrics and Gynecology*, XLVI (July, 1943), 38–52.
B. S. Burke, V. A. Beal, S. B. Kirkwood, and H. C. Stuart, "The Influence of Nutrition during Pregnancy upon the Condition of the Infant at Birth," *Journal of Nutrition*, XXVI (December, 1943), 569–83.

Nutrition and Health

women in the poorest diet group were in very poor physical condition at birth; that is, they were stillborn or died within a few days of birth, they were premature, had a serious congenital defect, or were immature in some way other than weight and length

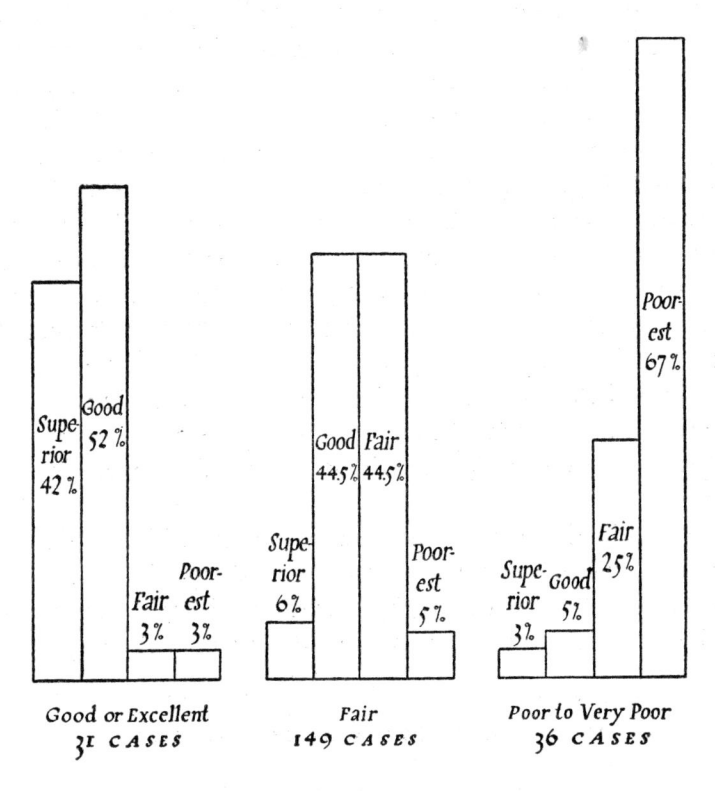

Good or Excellent	Fair	Poor to Very Poor
31 CASES	149 CASES	36 CASES
Superior 42%	Superior 6%	Superior 3%
Good 52%	Good 44.5%	Good 5%
Fair 3%	Fair 44.5%	Fair 25%
Poorest 3%	Poorest 5%	Poorest 67%

FIGURE I

RELATIONSHIP OF PRENATAL NUTRITION TO THE PHYSICAL CONDITION OF THE INFANT AT BIRTH AND WITHIN FIRST TWO WEEKS OF LIFE

(Courtesy of *Journal of Nutrition*, XXVI [December, 1943], 569)

alone. Another 25 percent of infants born to mothers in the poorest diet group were in only fair physical condition at birth. In other words, 92 percent of the women whose diets were very inadequate gave birth to infants who were in unsatisfactory condition. In this study all the stillborn infants, all except one of the neonatal deaths, all except one of the premature infants, and most of the infants with major congenital defects were born to women in the poorest diet group.

The over-all relationship found to exist between the physical condition of the infant at birth and the maternal diet is a highly significant one. Although it exists beyond any reasonable doubt, we are unable to explain the nature of this relationship or the manner in which it operates. I should like to emphasize, however, that the infants who were born in the poorest physical condition were almost exclusively confined to families in the poorest diet group. In this group the inadequacies in the diets were extreme, and no effort was made in the majority of cases to influence the woman to eat a better diet. It is likely, therefore, that in many instances the rating of the diet during pregnancy represents the woman's food habits for a considerable period of time previous to pregnancy. It seems probable that the mother's nutritional state at the time she enters pregnancy, as well as the quality and quantity of her diet during pregnancy, may be an important factor in determining the condition of the infant at birth.

The following table shows that the average birth weight and birth length of the infants born to mothers whose diets were good or excellent was 8 lbs., 8 oz., and their length 51.8 cm. (20.5 inches), in contrast to an average weight of 5 lbs., 13 oz. and

BIRTH WEIGHTS AND LENGTHS OF INFANTS GROUPED ACCORDING TO PRENATAL DIETARY RATING

	PRENATAL DIETARY RATING		
BIRTH WEIGHT *lbs.-oz.*	EXCELLENT OR GOOD	FAIR	POOR TO VERY POOR
Range	6-12 to 11-7	3-6 to 9-3	3-4 to 8-15
Average	8–8	7–7	5–13
BIRTH LENGTH *cm.*			
Average	51.8	50.0	47.2
Range	46.9 to 54.6	45.0 to 54.4	40.6 to 52.7

(Courtesy of *Journal of Nutrition*, XXVI [December, 1943], 569)

Nutrition and Health

length of 47.2 cm. (18.5 inches) for those infants whose mothers' diets were poor or very poor.

While no statistically significant relationship was found to exist between the diet during pregnancy and the length of labor of the women having their first baby, there were many more difficult types of delivery in the poorest diet group. This was true despite the fact that these infants averaged almost three pounds lighter in weight than the infants of mothers whose diets were good or excellent.

While we found also that a significant relationship existed between antepartum diet and complications of pregnancy (Fig. II), this relationship was less marked than that with the condition of the infant at birth.

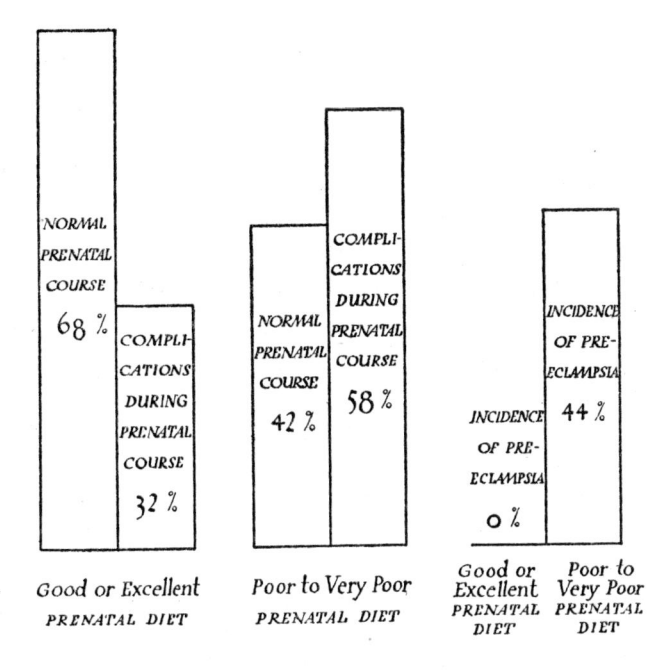

FIGURE II

RELATIONSHIP OF PRENATAL COURSE TO MOTHER'S DIET DURING PREGNANCY AND INCIDENCE OF PRE-ECLAMPSIA IN RELATION TO MOTHER'S DIET DURING PREGNANCY

(Courtesy of *American Journal of Obstetrics and Gynecology*, XLVI [July, 1943], 38)

If this is true, it is entirely possible that a woman may have an apparently satisfactory clinical course of pregnancy, but if her diet is sufficiently inadequate, the unborn baby may suffer. The relationship between the general dietary rating for pregnancy and the incidence of toxemia was also significant, although the number of cases was small. While there was no toxemia among the women whose diets were good or excellent, it developed in 8 percent (twelve cases) of the women whose diets were fair and in 44 percent (sixteen cases) of the women in the group with the poorest diets.

K. U. Toverud [10] has reported a study of approximately a thousand pregnant women in a special health district of Oslo who were given nutritional guidance during pregnancy as a part of prenatal care. Her results point to a relationship between maternal diet and the mother's health and course of pregnancy, as well as benefits to the newborn infant. The stillbirth rate in the supervised group for the years 1939–44 averaged 16 per 1,000 live births compared to 30 per 1,000 for the city of Oslo, while the neonatal death rate was 11 per 1,000 compared to 20.

Under the severe restrictions imposed by war, England appears to have profited considerably with respect to health as a result of her need to utilize all available food as efficiently as possible. Despite the monotony of the diet, the nutritional quality of the average English diet improved, especially in the lower income groups. Sir Wilson Jameson, of the British Ministry of Health,[11] and others [12] have pointed out that for the first time in the history of England special food, in the form of additional milk, eggs, supplementary vitamins, and other extra rations when possible, was made available to all pregnant women. The Ministry of Health and the Ministry of Foods instituted widespread propaganda programs for the use of these extra rations. A study of the stillbirth rates in England and Wales from 1928 through

[10] K. U. Toverud, *Beretning Om De Første 6 Ars Arbeid Ved Oslo Kommunes Helsestasjon For Mor Og Barn Pa Sagene* (1939–1944) (Oslo: Fabritius & Sønner, 1945), pp. 1–158.

[11] Wilson Jameson, "The Place of Nutrition in a Public Health Program," *American Journal of Public Health*, XXXVII (November, 1947), 1371–75.

[12] Ian Sutherland, "The Stillbirth-Rate in England and Wales in Relation to Social Influences," *Lancet*, II (December 28, 1946), 953–56.

Nutrition and Health

1944 showed that a sharp drop occurred in all counties following the institution of this rationing program. In the poorest economic districts the drop was greatest; in Wales it approximated 35 percent. The neonatal death rate and the prematurity rate have also declined, but to a lesser degree. The incidence of toxemia in England also fell following the institution of this program. These changes occurred when most conditions in England, other than nutrition, had deteriorated. Baird [13] has discussed the effect of these factors in Scotland and has stated that the stillbirth and neonatal death rates appear to be controlled by social conditions which operate through the mother. He emphasized that in England, Wales, and Scotland the stillbirth rate fell during the war period and that all age groups and parities were affected uniformly. All these workers have referred to the apparent operation of some factor on a national scale and considered it probable that improvement in the diets of the poorer women is the explanation.

Toxemia is one of the leading causes of death resulting from pregnancy, and it also is associated with a high incidence of premature births and a high infant mortality. The role of protein in relation to toxemia of pregnancy is still a debated problem. Strauss,[14] Arnell,[15] Tompkins,[16] and others have claimed a high incidence of toxemia among women on low-protein diets. As already stated, we found a significant relationship between the incidence of toxemia and the general rating of the antepartum diet. While the amount of protein in these diets was usually low, many other dietary essentials were also low, therefore it was not possible to conclude that protein was the sole dietary factor in-

---

[13] D. Baird, "Social Class and Foetal Mortality," *Lancet*, II (October 11, 1947), 531–35.

[14] M. B. Strauss, "Observations on Etiology of Toxemias of Pregnancy: IV. Primary Role of Plasma Proteins in Conditioning Water Retention and Edema Formation in Normal and Toxemic Pregnancy," *American Journal of Medical Sciences*, CXCV (June, 1938), 723–28.

[15] R. E. Arnell, D. W. Goldman, and F. J. Bertucci, "Protein Deficiencies in Pregnancy," *Journal of the American Medical Association*, CXXVII (April 28, 1945), 1101–07.

[16] W. T. Tompkins, "The Significance of Nutritional Deficiency in Pregnancy; a Preliminary Report," *Journal of the International College of Surgeons*, IV (April, 1941), 147–54.

volved. In other studies already mentioned the incidence of toxemia decreased with an improved dietary intake. While there is still controversy among well-informed individuals concerning the cause of toxemia, it is generally accepted that a high-protein diet does not predispose to the condition, and the major weight of evidence would seem to indicate that toxemia occurs more often among chronically malnourished women than among well-nourished women and that protein is one of the factors most frequently deficient. In fact, there is positive evidence to justify the recommendation of a diet high in protein, especially during the latter part of pregnancy. The well-known nitrogen balance studies of Macy, Hunscher, and others [17] have shown that women normally store relatively large amounts of protein during pregnancy over and above that needed by the fetus and accessory structures. These metabolic studies indicate that a protein requirement of 845 to 900 gm. (135 to 145 gm. nitrogen) above the woman's maintenance requirement is representative of the total net requirement for the fetus and its accessory structures. Under favorable circumstances, the pregnant woman retains an additional 1,250 to 2,500 gm. of protein (200 to 400 gm. nitrogen) as a safety factor in preparation for delivery and for lactation. These figures represent an increased requirement of 10 to 20 gm. of protein daily during the latter months of pregnancy.

We [18] have shown that when the pregnant woman consumes less than 75 gm. of protein daily during the latter part of pregnancy her infant tends to be short and light in weight and is likely to receive a low pediatric rating in other respects. We have also demonstrated [19] that high-protein and high-calcium intakes dur-

[17] I. G. Macy and H. A. Hunscher, "Evaluation of Maternal Nitrogen and Mineral Needs during Embryonic and Infant Development," *American Journal of Obstetrics and Gynecology*, XXVII (June, 1934), 878–88.

[18] B. S. Burke, V. V. Harding, and H. C. Stuart, "Nutrition Studies during Pregnancy: IV. Relation of Protein Content of Mother's Diet during Pregnancy to Birth Length, Birth Weight and Condition of Infant at Birth," *Journal of Pediatrics*, XXIII (November, 1943), 506–15.

[19] H. C. Stuart, "Findings on Examinations of Newborn Infants and Infants during the Neonatal Period Which Appear to Have a Relationship to the Diets of Their Mothers during Pregnancy," *Federation Proceedings*, IV (September, 1945), 271–81.

Nutrition and Health

ing the latter months of pregnancy seem to be associated with better than average osseous development at birth, and that when the diet of the mother is poor in these important nutrients osseous development tends to be retarded.

We realize fully that nutrition is but one of the many environmental factors which may affect the mother and her infant during pregnancy, but there now appears to be strong evidence that good diet during pregnancy lessens the likelihood of complications and contributes to a safer delivery. The evaluation of nutritional status and the giving of dietary advice to every woman as a part of routine prenatal care would seem, therefore, to be amply justified. The added evidence that women who have good or excellent diets during pregnancy are much more likely to have healthy, well-developed infants and much less likely to have stillborn or prematurely born infants, or infants who die in the neonatal period, increases the incentive to improve maternal dietaries.

We have referred to what was accomplished in England and Wales during the war in the reduction of the incidence of stillbirths. The stillbirth rate in this country is known to be higher with the advancing order of births, and to be relatively high among mothers who bear a large number of children in rapid succession.[20] The evidence suggests that nutritional depletion may play a large part in bringing about this result.

Let us now consider briefly what a concerted effort in this country to improve the nutrition of the pregnant woman might accomplish in the reduction of infant mortality. The remarkable reduction that has already been accomplished is well known. In "Frontiers of Human Welfare" [21] one is reminded that in New York City about the middle of the nineteenth century the infant death rate was 275 per 1,000 live births, largely from preventable causes, while today it is only 28. The National Office of Vital Statistics of the United States Public Health Service [22] has re-

---

[20] "Current Comment: 'Stillbirths,'" *Journal of the American Medical Association*, CXXXVI (February 21, 1948), 558.
[21] *Frontiers in Human Welfare* (New York: Community Service Society, 1948).
[22] "Miscellany: 'Infant Mortality,'" *Journal of the American Medical Association*, CXXXVI (February 14, 1948), 492.

cently released a summary on infant mortality in the United States for 1945. The figure given for the country as a whole is 38.3 deaths per 1,000 live births as compared to 99.9 deaths per 1,000 live births in 1915. A study of the figures shows that most of the reduction has been among infants over one month of age. The decrease for the age group from six to eleven months was 80 percent, and that for one to six months 70 percent, while under one month it was 45 percent, and under one day only 25 percent. More infant deaths now occur under one month of age than during the remainder of infant life. Thus, neonatal mortality constitutes a decidedly greater proportion of total infant deaths than formerly, and mortality during the first day of life is now extremely high in comparison with each of the other age groups. A preponderance of the deaths from premature birth, congenital malformations, and injury at birth occurs during the neonatal period, and more than half of the deaths from premature birth and injury at birth occur during the first day of life. The report states that improved conditions of public health and advances in medical knowledge with regard to problems of infant disease and death have resulted in a tremendous reduction in mortality during later infancy. They call attention to the fact that, while much room for improvement in postnatal care still remains, major progress in the future must come through improvement of the prenatal and early extra-uterine environment.

No one has as yet demonstrated a statistically significant relationship between nutrition and congenital malformations in human beings. In our study [23] the major number of infants with congenital defects were born to women in the group with the poorest maternal diet, but the number is too small to be significant. Warkany,[24] however, has demonstrated beyond any reasonable doubt that certain congenital malformations in animals result when riboflavin is deficient in the maternal diet. He also has demonstrated congenital malformations of the eye as a result of vitamin A deficiency during pregnancy, and another syndrome

[23] Burke, Beal, Kirkwood, and Stuart, *American Journal of Obstetrics and Gynecology*, loc. cit.
[24] J. Warkany, "Congenital Malformations Induced by Maternal Nutritional Deficiency," *Journal of Pediatrics*, XXV (December, 1944), 476–80.

Nutrition and Health

of congenital malformations due to vitamin D deficiency in the mother. I mention this because, if Warkany's findings in relation to congenital malformations in animals should prove to be, even in part, applicable to human beings, it would be futile to correct the maternal diet after the third month of pregnancy in an attempt to prevent congenital anomalies. If the maternal nutritional state is a factor in their causation, then the mother's diet must be improved and maintained satisfactorily during early pregnancy.

Present knowledge as it relates to pregnancy certainly justifies a concerted effort on the part of all obstetricians, general practitioners, and persons and agencies concerned with the health and welfare of the families of this nation to see that the mother of the family has a proper diet at all times, and that when she is pregnant extra effort be made to see that she has a diet suited to her needs from the time of her child's conception. This should be determined by a dietary history of her usual food habits and an evaluation of her nutritional state. It is necessary that she understand the importance of such a diet to her own health and to her unborn child in order that she be motivated to carry out the instructions given her as completely as possible. Such dietary instruction must be adjusted to her own food habits, likes and dislikes, economic status, and mode of life. If her family budget does not permit the necessary foods, some means should be found to supplement her diet to the proper level. Three considerations are important in any forward-looking program for improving maternal nutrition: (1) special nutrition services should be provided in connection with all prenatal clinics and other organized maternal care services; (2) the private obstetrician must, obviously, offer the same type of nutrition service as that which should be given in all prenatal clinics; if he cannot render this service himself, he should be able to call upon a suitably trained nutritionist; (3) sound health education should be taught young women in high school, in college, and in industry. Education of this type should also be arranged for young married women and their husbands and for those who are contemplating marriage. Such courses should stress, not only normal nutrition, but the special nutritional requirements that are imposed by pregnancy.

While I have chosen to devote the major part of this discussion to the benefits which might accrue to future generations through a concentrated effort to improve the nutritional state of the childbearing women of this nation, I am not unmindful that the children of today will be the parents of tomorrow's families. Nutrition is one of the most important of the complex and interrelated factors which exert profound effects upon the growth and development of the child between birth and maturity. It is only by the use of a combination of clinical and biochemical techniques together with a detailed dietary history that we can evaluate a child's progress in growth and development and health from the standpoint of nutrition.

Biochemical techniques have enabled us also to increase our knowledge of the nutritional value of human milk. In recommending breast milk for today's infant, we have sound knowledge of the nutritional value of colostrum and mature human milk, due to the extensive studies of Macy and her co-workers.[25] Maynard and his co-workers [26] have compared cow's milk with human milk in nutritional value. Our knowledge of the composition of human milk, and of the other benefits which breast feeding gives, is such today, that we can with conviction urge every mother who is well-nourished to make every possible effort to give her child this advantage.

If for any reason an infant cannot be breast fed, two points deserve special consideration. When cow's milk is used in the feeding mixture, it is necessary to supply approximately twice as much protein per unit of body weight as the corresponding amount of breast milk furnishes. (This means that the infant fed cow's milk should receive approximately 4 gm. of protein per kilogram of body weight.) Unless this amount of protein is sup-

[25] I. G. Macy, H. H. Williams, J. P. Pratt, and B. M. Hamil, "Human Milk Studies: XIX et seq. Implications of Breast Feeding and Their Investigation," American Journal of Diseases of Children, LXX (September, 1945), 135–41.

[26] J. M. Lawrence, B. L. Herrington, and L. A. Maynard, "Human Milk Studies: XXVII. Comparative Values of Bovine and Human Milks in Infant Feeding," American Journal of Diseases of Children, LXX (September, 1945), 193–99.

plied, Jeans [27] points out, the artificially fed baby has poorer muscles and poorer motor development than the breast-fed infant. Secondly, if an infant must be artificially fed, it is important that he enjoy, as nearly as possible, the same feeling of security as the breast-fed baby. Another important consideration in the successful handling of an infant's feeding schedule is the fact that good pediatric advice recommends that an infant be nursed whenever he indicates that he is hungry. As a matter of fact, a baby who is allowed to choose his own feeding schedule usually adjusts to a normal routine within a short space of time.[28] A feeding schedule of this nature gives direct gratification to the basic hunger urge and possibly avoids feeding difficulties and other maladjustments of later childhood.

The successful feeding of a child as he approaches the end of his first year must consider his appetite in relation to his rate of growth. The very rapid growth rate of infancy slows, and with it comes a normal lessening of appetite. Between one and two years of age the child becomes more interested in the world around him. He is less interested in his food, and while the total amount of what he eats may be somewhat greater than in infancy, his caloric requirement per unit of body weight has decreased. Many feeding problems could be avoided if this information were made a routine part of our feeding instructions. Since this lack of interest in food is natural and may continue throughout much of the preschool period it is necessary that a child's food be selected primarily to furnish the essential growth constituents. When the diet includes the recommended allowances of these constituents, sufficient calories are usually supplied. Many low-protein diets are encountered in this period. This is especially true when a child has been allowed to eat foods which are primarily high in carbohydrate.

Attention should be given to the fact that when energy needs are inadequately supplied, protein will be used for energy and

[27] P. C. Jeans, "The Feeding of Healthy Infants and Children," *Journal of the American Medical Association*, CXX (November 21, 1942), 913–21.
[28] C. A. Aldrich and E. S. Hewitt, "A Self-regulating Feeding Program for Infants," *Journal of the American Medical Association*, CXXXV (October 11, 1947), 340–42.

growth may suffer. When, as is the case in many of the devastated areas of Europe and Asia, the caloric intake is very deficient and the protein content of the diet is also low, growth is seriously impaired.[29] A child who is fed such an inadequate diet is short, light in weight, his general physical appearance is poor, he has poor muscles, and his bones are usually small and light. He is often quiet and listless and lacks that sparkle and animal spirit which radiate from a well-nourished child. These findings have been substantiated by our work with a small series of similar children who were referred to the pediatric department of the Massachusetts General Hospital.[30]

Adolescence is another neglected and little understood period. In this period the requirements for all the nutritional essentials are increased just prior to and during the adolescent growth spurt. Many of the children included in our study of growth and development are now in the adolescent age range, and while we are not able to draw any definite conclusions as yet, because so many factors are involved, it seems apparent that nutrition has played an important part in the determination of the growth and general well-being of these children. It is our belief that the child's food habits will be no better than those of his family. If we are to improve the food habits of the children, therefore, we must improve the family pattern of eating.

[29] H. C. Stuart, "Effects of Protein Deficiency on the Pregnant Woman and Fetus and on the Infant and Child," *New England Journal of Medicine*, CCXXXVI (April 3, 1947), 507-13; CCXXXVI (April 10, 1947), 537-41.

[30] N. B. Talbot, H. E. Sobel, B. S. Burke, E. Lindemann, and S. B. Kaufman, "Dwarfism in Healthy Children: Its Possible Relation to Emotional, Nutritional and Endocrine Disturbances," *New England Journal of Medicine*, CCXXXVI (May 22, 1947), 783-93.

Nutrition in the Home and in the Community

CHARLES GLEN KING

RECENT DISCOVERIES in nutrition research and practice have high-lighted the fact that in human nutrition we should be more mindful of the phrase, "In the beginning . . ." Possibly some devotees of science and sociology would be slow to identify the source book for the above phrase, but they should be informed that even in those early days, the man had only a weak excuse when a mistake was brought to light in the use of food. The modern Adam cannot take refuge in the Biblical precedent of putting all the responsibility on Eve; he could be challenged with the gentle suggestion that if he had provided an orange instead of an apple of unknown vitamin A and C content, little Cain might have become a better citizen.

How are we to accomplish good nutrition in American homes and communities?

First, we must establish assurance that the goal is worth fighting for. Secondly, the knowledge that good nutrition, in contrast to a full stomach, is an inescapable and major factor in human health should be taught as early as spelling and arithmetic. And it should be taught with as much conviction. It should be set forth so clearly that an intelligent response would be nearly automatic. We need to recognize, however, that both the scientific evidence and the techniques of education call for some revision with the years or they lose their effectiveness.

It is a challenge to those who are concerned with the practical aspects of nutrition to incorporate into attractive meals both a sense of enjoyment, in terms of appearance, flavor, and environment, and a valid sense of satisfaction in a long-time perspective. Good food can taste good, whatever you may think of liver and spinach, and it is improved by a sense of humor. But in nutrition, as in morals, the use of short cuts instead of discipline increases the risk of tragedy.

Those who have read Arnold Joseph Toynbee's recent book, *A Study of History*, are likely to remember two dominant ideas: one deals with the great role played by successive challenges and response in human development; and a second is concerned with the requirement of a cohesive ideal to guide human behavior. Both these factors are constantly at play in the current world food situation. We can see them as we focus the microscope of current experience to examine each individual nation, community, home, and individual.

There are serious challenges to progress in terms of health, convenience, cost, education, and research. Nor will we solve the problems without vigorous, unselfish service. The family physician, the public health officer, Red Cross teachers, schoolteachers, social service workers, heads of families, nurses, restaurant managers, grocerymen, and food manufacturers should have an active interest in preventing the waste in human health that results from poor nutrition.

The sociologist and the head of a family will sense quickly the connotations implied by the statement that "a house does not make a home." Less obvious, but quite as true, is the statement, "Enough to eat does not mean enough to nourish." As chemists study the composition of foods and explore with medical scientists the complex relationships of food to health, the more certain it is that current food practices need to be improved.

Let me cite a few illustrations from recent progress:

1. From studies of tooth decay, both in children and in animals, it is clear that one of the most important factors in protecting the teeth is the diet of the mother. How much of the story is told in the time before the young are born, as differentiated from the nursing period, remains to be discovered. But no longer should there be any doubt that food practices are at the root of the tooth problem.

2. Many leading physicians and nutrition scientists are convinced that when an infant is not breast fed, there is a sacrifice of nutritional quality in its diet. The chemical evidence is very clear regarding differences in the composition of cow's milk compared to human milk. In addition to the chemical problem, there is an apparent risk psychologically for both the mother and the infant. But several generations may come and go before we have an adequate appraisal of the effects of differing food intakes on health and personality. I hope there may be recognized in this picture a basis for my earlier reference to the value of challenge and response and a sense of idealism in human society. A safe public milk supply has contributed to a great improvement in infant and child health, but there is need for caution against going too far in the direction of formula feeding when it is not necessary—and usually it is not necessary in early infancy.

3. New vitamins are being discovered year after year, and several of them are known to be easily destroyed. There is an obvious need to emphasize shorter cooking time and to give more attention to high-quality, fresh foods. Vitamins B_6, C, B_1, and B_c (folic acid) are good examples of essential nutrients that are easily destroyed. They are present in fresh meats, fresh fruits, and in green leafy vegetables, but like some folks' tempers, there is a limit to their endurance. When these nutrients are gone for a time from the family table, there follows insidiously, loss of radiant complexions, anemia, distorted bone marrow, poor appetites, and lowered protection against infections.

4. Dr. Edward Park's report, based upon many years of careful study at the Johns Hopkins Hospital, stated that about one third to one half of the children who came to autopsy there showed evidence of injury to the bony structures, caused by malnutrition. This was true despite the fact that in almost none of these cases had there been a diagnosis of nutritional deficiencies. Again, Dr. Frederick Tisdall reported that in Toronto, 50 percent of the cases of infant scurvy sent into the hospital in recent years had not been properly diagnosed before arrival. The physicians who are closest to the problem recognize the need for better means of identifying the less severe forms of malnutrition.

5. The New York Public Health Research Institute has made an outstanding contribution to the techniques of detecting malnutrition in children of school age. The demonstration by this group that one can gain a reasonably accurate and reliable appraisal of nutritional status by chemical analysis of a few drops of blood taken from a fingertip has opened up a new chapter in public health nutrition. Such chemical analyses will not replace the physician or substitute for his role in making a physical examination and diagnosis, nor will they replace the need for diet records. But they will greatly facilitate the problem of getting exact evidence of the kind of food practices that are at fault in a given community or in an individual patient. Corrective and preventive measures will then be possible without waiting to find severe forms of malnutrition, such as scurvy and rickets. For example, with samples taken at the rate of about one per minute, from school groups, the Institute was able to report accurately on the blood concentration of iron, protein, the red blood pigment (hemoglobin), vitamin A, carotene, vitamin C, and phosphatase (in order to detect rickets). It is now possible to add a test for vitamin B_1 and vitamin B_2 to the list of measurements, and still use only a few drops of blood from a fingertip.

As an example of the practical results to be gained from such surveys, the Institute's research workers were able to demonstrate that in a particular school group with a favorable educational and economic background, the intake of vitamin C was relatively satisfactory, whereas in another, it was definitely low even though there was no evidence of scurvy in the classical sense. A situation of that kind can be corrected with additions to the diet of citrus fruit, tomatoes, cabbage, or broccoli, as the families may prefer. Basically, the problem is not a matter of income; it is a matter of education. Similar contrasts were found in regard to the consumption of green leafy vegetables, as reflected in vitamin A and carotene analyses. In another school, there was a considerable amount of anemia. They were able to screen out the individuals in whom a simple iron deficiency had caused a poor blood supply. Curative measures were then specific and immediately effective.

6. Another study in the New York area, conducted by Professor

Henry C. Sherman and his associates at Columbia University, has given concrete evidence of the long-term significance of food habits. The data show unmistakably that gains in health through a wise choice of foods can be achieved well above the levels of nutrition that result in immediate evidence of suppressed growth or injury.

7. After more than one hundred years of chemical studies on proteins, we are just reaching the point where proteins and their fragments, the amino acids, can be used or interpreted in human feeding, on a scientific basis. Since 1942 the human tests have almost caught up with the rat tests. By itself, this would represent a limited goal, but the limitations are shattered when we see the resultant discoveries reaching out into the zones where scientists are in a better position to fight cancer, infections, kidney disease, liver disease, surgical shock, starvation, anemia, diabetes, and muscular weakness.

One cannot read current research reports and fail to be impressed by the need for far greater care in teaching children and adults to use foods in a more reasonable way. If the term "health" is too vague or in danger of being overworked, a valid, forthright claim can be made from the point of view of athletic development, which appeals to nearly every boy and to many girls. An honest appeal can also be made on more aesthetic grounds, on the basis of social attainment, graceful carriage, and skin glamour, which I am told appeal to some girls, that is, when they are very young. Among adults, the argument that proper nutrition will postpone the day when health will break can command strong evidence, in terms of such common conditions as hardened arteries, high blood pressure, unstable nerves, and skin that has aged prematurely.

We could scarcely have a more impressive record of the importance of simple improvements in food practices than we have had from Great Britain during and since the war. Despite an initial rise in maternal and infant death rates in the 1940–41 period, within the first year of launching a vigorous nutrition education and feeding program, the British were able to lower the maternal and infant death rates to all-time low values, and to continue this progressive improvement each year through 1946. By 1945, they could also cite a lowered incidence of tuberculosis and of dental caries.

We have had a similar trend in the United States, but the evidence is not quite so clear in relating the gains in health specifically to improvements in nutrition. In Norway, again, the record is valid and impressive, in that the rate of dental caries among preschool and school children dropped about 65 percent during the war period. Their best dental authorities (e.g., Dean G. Toverud, of the University School of Dentistry) are confident that the major cause of the gain was the improvement in eating habits. The dental situation in the United States at the beginning of the war has been dramatically summarized by one of the medical officers in the cryptic statement that in order to get enough men for the armed forces, the dental standard was lowered to a basic requirement of two jaws.

Sir John Boyd Orr has told of the great gains made in industrial feeding early in the British experiences of the second World War. Industrial unrest in individual manufacturing plants frequently yielded to a common-sense provision for eating lunch in dining rooms that were more aesthetic than a greasy aisle beside noisy machinery, and where there was at least a possibility of having something hot. In the field of human relations, many leaders in industry have a great opportunity to improve the health of their employees, as well as to foster a better feeling toward management, by giving more attention to industrial feeding.

There is a tendency to be complacent about food in America, just because a home or a community does not have a constant threat of pellagra, rickets, or gross hunger. We should aim at levels of nutrition that are distinctly above those characterized by deficiency diseases. This does not mean gorging ourselves with food. Quite the contrary! It means teaching every child and adult not to eat too much, but to be consistent in consuming foods of assured nutritive quality: citrus fruits and juices or tomatoes, as one type; green leafy foods that are not overcooked, as a second type; milk, meat, fish, cheese, and eggs, in a third group; whole or enriched cereals, as a fourth type; and fifth, a sufficient amount of energy foods, in the form of fats, starches, and sugars, to keep going at full steam without accumulating excess body weight. It is stylish and technically correct not to be fat.

Any adult can find convincing evidence that excessive body weight means a greater risk of such conditions as diabetes, high blood pressure, hardening of the arteries, heart failure, cancer, and a shortened life span. For example, the data compiled by the Metropolitan Life Insurance Company [1] show that among men who are 25 percent or more above normal body weight, the death rate rises far above normal; the death rate from diabetes, specifically, is eight times higher than among persons of average weight and thirteen times higher than in underweight persons. High blood pressure is found to be twice as common in obese men as in average-weight men. On the other hand, when body weight is distinctly below normal, the death rate from tuberculosis rises sharply.

In contrast to the problem of calories, a departure from good nutrition practice in regard to vitamins, minerals, and proteins is difficult to identify or measure. The resultant symptoms tend to vary in different persons, and, furthermore, the development of symptoms usually requires months or even years.

The family dinner table involves much more than nutrition. It should be a place of inspiration and enjoyment, not a place of punishment. The quirks and cynicism of parents at the table can cause more than malnutrition in children. One of the most difficult problems that I encountered in working with students was raised by a very intelligent senior who was fighting within himself, not only against going into professional scientific work that dealt with food, but even against marrying and building a home. The difficulty arose primarily because, to quote him, "Every dollar that my mother spent was fought over at the family dinner table."

In contrast, consistent discipline at the dinner table can have a carry-over value in character-building that is perhaps as important as good teeth and good muscles. For example, I have

---

[1] Courtesy of Louis I. Dublin, M.D., in charge of Health and Welfare Division of the Metropolitan Life Insurance Company.

known families that had practically no trouble in getting children to eat everything on their plates by uniformly requiring, without argument, that the main course must be finished or "there will be no dessert." As a logical result there was no nagging, few heartaches, and very few stomach-aches.

The family table is not exactly a chapel, but within the family unit it can, and should, be almost as inspirational.

The Harvard School of Public Health has made an excellent contribution to the techniques of education through the elementary grades and high school. Their leaflet, "Goals for Nutrition Education," provides a well-organized approach at successive grade levels through the elementary and secondary schools. We need more emphasis upon this kind of approach.

School lunches represent another valuable opportunity for education in the science of nutrition. There are difficulties in regard to the economic aspects of such a program, but the side issues regarding policies and cost should not be permitted to submerge the major issue of making food available to growing children and the accompanying opportunity for sound education. To cite a specific problem, school lunches should not serve primarily as a means of removing surplus products from the market place (as they have in many communities), nor should pressure groups be permitted to push their individual interests into an area where the child's health should be paramount.

It is not enough to note that our food picture is more favorable than that in the Philippine Islands, for example, where the causes of death are currently listed in this order: (1) tuberculosis; (2) beriberi; (3) malaria; and (4) gastrointestinal diseases. We should do much better here and help them much more. Where is the logic of wasting both our health and our abundant food supply, for lack of education, while half the world struggles against the risk of tuberculosis and famine?

It would be difficult to picture a single measure that would make a greater contribution to raising American standards of living, or a greater contribution to the enjoyment of life, than would result from an effective nutrition program. It is worth the effort, and the world calls for our response.

Food for the Family of Nations

F. VERZÁR

As a member of the Food and Agriculture Organization of the United Nations, I would like to outline briefly the activities of the FAO, for it is our aim to make the family of nations a force for peace by fighting hunger and malnutrition.

Our purpose is to prepare for prosperity with the aid of an equilibrium between production and consumption, to eliminate the basis of difficulties which can lead to troubles in the family of nations. It is a commonplace, but too often not a joke, that in family life the way to the heart is through the stomach, and it is a fact that in an astonishing number of cases in the divorce courts the complaint concerns poor housekeeping and cooking. It is hunger in the life of nations which is far too often a source of unrest.

When and how has nutrition come into the problems of world politics?

Physiology, the science of the functions of our body, had for a long time not realized the primary importance of nutrition in all body functions. Until about 1900 not much more than the quantity of food, measured in calories, and the quantity of proteins, without regard to their origin, were studied. Nothing was understood about the importance of the quality of food, especially of the so-called "accessory" food factors. It is true that about 1840 the famous French physiologist François Magendie recognized that a dog cannot be kept alive on sugar alone; we might also cite a series of British naval experiences, going back as far as the seventeenth century, when scurvy was fought with fresh fruit, and to the experiences in the Japanese Navy about 1870 when beriberi was abolished with a change of the food ration from pure rice to rice with meat. It was about 1880 that Gustav Bunge gave to one of his pupils the problem of finding out whether a natural food such as milk has the same value as its purified constituents. They showed that a mouse could grow normally on milk but that this would no longer be the case if the animal were fed the purified protein, fat, sugar, and salts of the milk. However, it was not recognized at that time what factors were responsible for such an important difference. Another thirty years elapsed before it was understood that there are accessory food factors, which in 1911, and thereafter, were called vitamins.

I myself am a theoretical physiologist who has spent all his life on so-called "fundamental research," that is, on problems of the functions of the organs of the body. Such work may seem to be far from practical, but without such work not one step could have been taken in modern food research and food economics.

In times of social and economic stability, one can serve theoretical fundamental research without asking for its practical application. But our times are different. With the quick change of conditions of human life through new technical knowledge, new ways of communication, and through better hygienic conditions, leading to great increases of population, living conditions have changed so much that science has the obligation to find ways of adaptation. At the present time, coördination of scientific knowledge with practical methods of influencing the life of the peoples is an absolute necessity.

After the first World War, the League of Nations took steps to organize medical, hygienic, and nutritional knowledge, and to correlate this with agricultural and technical production all over the world. The years after the first World War created, especially in Europe, formidable nutrition problems. The depression of the 1930s added new problems throughout the world.

It was at that time clearly recognized that even in a peacefully advancing country, such as the United Kingdom, a great part of the population, actually more than half, was not fed optimally, not even sufficiently. A famous book, *Food, Health and Income*, by Sir John Boyd Orr, then Director of the Rowett Research In-

Food for the Family of Nations

stitute in Aberdeen, Scotland, called attention to these facts. The eyes of the public and of some officials were opened to these new problems of nutrition as a factor in public health and happiness.

In 1935, at the proposal of the Australian delegation, the Assembly of the League of Nations placed nutrition on its program, and a beginning was made on the international plans to correlate nutrition, health, agriculture, and economic policy. It is worth noting that the League committee on nutrition reported to the Assembly that, "The malnutrition which exists in all countries is at once a challenge and an opportunity: a challenge to men's consciences and an opportunity to eradicate a social evil by methods which will increase economic prosperity."

Since the second World War this work has been taken up on a much larger scale by the Food and Agriculture Organization of the United Nations. The FAO was conceived at the Hot Springs Conference in 1943, where an interim commission was formed. It is a specialized agency of the United Nations, just as are the International Labor Office, the World Health Organization, the United Nations Educational, Scientific and Cultural Organization, the International Bank for Reconstruction and Development, and the International Monetary Fund.

The constitution of the FAO was drafted at its first session in Quebec, 1945, when Sir John Boyd Orr was appointed Director-General. By the terms of its charter, the FAO has two main purposes: to banish hunger and malnutrition from the world, and to help bring prosperity and stability to agriculture.

The general objectives of the long-range program of the FAO as stated at the second session of the annual conference of the FAO in Copenhagen in 1946 are: development and organization of production, distribution, and utilization of basic foods to provide diets on a health standard for the people of all countries; and stabilization of agricultural prices at levels fair to producers and consumers alike. Such efforts cannot be limited to the agricultural field, but have been related to expanding world economy. An essential part of general development is the widespread application of advanced agricultural techniques. Special problems arise as to the instability of supplies and prices of agricultural commodities. International arrangements were proposed which deal with stocks, ranges of international prices, export shares in the world market, means to extend consumption, and ways to stabilize prices at fair levels.

At the foundation of the FAO, the United Nations Relief and Rehabilitation Administration was thought to be able to accomplish the immediate postwar relief and rehabilitation tasks. It was not understood at that time that not only war destruction, but also the low productivity of many densely populated areas of the world, would prolong food scarcity for an increasing world population. Thus the world became more interested in immediate food relief for densely populated Europe and Asia than in the long-term problems for which the FAO originally planned a program.

In May, 1946, the FAO, therefore, called the special Washington meeting on urgent food problems. Here the International Emergency Food Council was created, which had to survey needs and available supplies of food and also to allocate certain necessities of production, such as fertilizers, etc. A number of special committees of experts transmitted its recommendations to member nations.

In August, 1947, the third session of the annual conference of the FAO was held in Geneva, and again the FAO realized the necessity of helping to alleviate the serious food scarcity throughout the world. It was this rather than the long-term agricultural improvement program which was discussed in Geneva. Fifty-four countries were present, represented by their high officials, which indicated the interest which nations were taking in the FAO and its work. The discussions integrated the diverse national programs to a common attack, and finally a World Food Council (a council of the FAO) was constituted to act between the sessions of the annual conference. It consists of eighteen member governments which have to keep the changing world food situation under constant review.

The Geneva conference stated: "Considering the food supply as a whole, the decline in cereal supplies will much more than offset the increases in supplies of other foods." The consequent

Food for the Family of Nations 233

shortages and famine prevailing in certain countries will cause further mortality and jeopardize the physical development of the younger generation. Indeed, such conditions may sharpen or even provoke social unrest in countries where reasonable levels of standards are not yet enjoyed. They can easily be contributory to international disorder or even to armed conflict. It stated further: "The longer range prospects are not promising. The output of nutritional desirable foods, such as milk, meat and eggs will increase only slowly."

Present consumption levels are in many countries, or in parts of their population, considerably below prewar levels, but even before the war there was much undernutrition and malnutrition, and food supplies never met the needs of the populations in quantity or in quality. The present grave food crisis is likely to continue in an acute form for at least two years. It will require excellent harvests in all the main producing areas in 1949 to bring the acute stage of the crisis to an end, and world-wide bounteous harvests in any one year are improbable.

Once this acute stage is over, it is rather probable that the world will find itself in a subacute stage of food shortage which will be sustained by three different factors:

1. Population growth is a problem in many parts of the world. In India between 1931 and 1941 the rate of increase was 1.4 percent per year, an increase of 50,000,000 people in ten years. In Java, the Philippines, Formosa, and Siam this rate is even exceeded. No reliable figures are available for China.

The increasing crude birth rate in Western Europe and North America increased greatly after the second World War. In the first half of 1947, compared with the period from 1937 to 1939, the increase was 45 percent in the United Kingdom, 46 percent in France, 40 percent in the Netherlands, and 50 percent in the United States. While these rates will probably not be maintained, the decrease of infant mortality in many countries acts in the same direction. The number of children will remain high for some time. It has been calculated that in the United States in 1937–39 there were 2,500,000, and in 1947 there were about 4,000,000 children one year of age.

2. An increasing demand for food will add to the food shortage. This is the result of the national policies in all advanced countries, designed to maintain full employment. This demand is directed especially toward the more expensive animal products. Economic prosperity always increases the consumption of these foods, and the demand could, therefore, increase in the coming years.

3. A more equitable distribution of foodstuffs adds to a certain food shortage. It is also the policy of advanced nations, and it is the result of nutritional knowledge that many governments learned during the war, to insure a more equitable sharing of food supplies, especially those of special nutritional value. For this purpose one has markedly to increase food consumption in the lower income groups. If the national food situation requires a careful husbanding of resources, this can only be carried out by decreasing the food consumption of the better income groups.

A famous example in recent years is the United Kingdom, where the normal consumer was allowed only three pints of milk per week, two ounces of cheese, and one shilling's worth of meat, less than half the prewar normal consumption of the well-to-do groups. But all children now have their milk ration, and one obvious result is that the growth and weight of children in all classes are approximately the same, in contrast to prewar days when there was a marked difference in weight and height between the children of the wealthy class and those of the poorer class. In spite of this, the consumption of fluid milk in the United Kingdom is now 45 percent higher than before the war, 4 percent higher for cheese, and only 9 percent less for meat. We may be pretty sure that the consumers' demand will remain at this level in the lower income groups and will probably increase again in the higher income groups.

At present, the FAO functions temporarily in Washington. In October, 1947, there were 174 technically qualified workers and a staff of about 380. Since the highest standards of efficiency and technical competence are considered of paramount importance in the FAO, our staff members are appointed in accordance with

Food for the Family of Nations

those criteria, and selected on as wide a geographical basis as is possible. In the nutrition division thirteen countries are represented among 17 workers. Yet these employees do not officially represent in any sense the countries from which they come. Their responsibilities are exclusively international in character. They do not receive instructions in regard to the discharge of their duties from any authority external to the organization. The staff members are expected to divest themselves as far as is humanly possible of national interests and become members of a world service.

The FAO is built up of technical divisions in six fields—agriculture; nutrition; fisheries; forestry; economics, marketing and statistics; and rural welfare. For each technical division there is a standing advisory committee to consider the more technical aspects of the work. The committee for the Nutrition Division consists of a group of fourteen internationally known workers in the field of nutrition. Its chairman is the well-known British physician Lord Horder.

The Agriculture Division has as its primary task assisting member governments to improve agricultural production in their countries. This is done by providing the technical agriculturists for formal missions, sending specialists to help deal with specific problems, convening meetings of technical workers to develop solutions to problems that affect more than one country, aiding governments in preparing development plans, finding specialists whom the governments can employ on such projects, and conducting and publishing results of studies aimed at the solution of important agricultural problems. Particular attention is being given to irrigation, drainage, farm machinery and implements, fertilizers, control of infestation of stored food products, control of animal diseases—particularly those, such as rinderpest, which require international action—soil conservation, bettering production through the use of improved varieties of plants and types of animals, and finding ways of increasing the production of meat and milk in areas where the human diet is deficient in animal protein.

The Fisheries Division studies the great possibilities for increasing human food through fishing. It plans coöperation for uniformity in, and improvement of, fisheries statistics. It publishes commodity studies on salted and other fish products and serves as a clearinghouse for technical knowledge which makes for improvement in quality.

The Forestry and Forestry Production Division organized in 1947 a regional meeting for Europe to exchange information on short- and long-range forestry and forest products problems and plans. From this have resulted effective relations with the Economic Commission for Europe and establishment of a forestry working group in Europe. In 1949 the World Silviculture Congress will be held in Finland. Advance studies of a possible Far East Forestry and Forestry Products Conference in 1949 are under way.

The Division of Economics, Marketing, and Statistics assists through working out for member governments standard procedures for the development and improvement of statistical services relating to food and agriculture. It helps to establish in different countries production targets for food and other agricultural products, as a basis for organization of production and as a guide to intelligent international consultation. It takes into account nutritional requirements, national and international market outlook, and the conservation and efficient use of agricultural resources.

While the whole of the FAO is concerned with rural welfare, with bettering the conditions of life of country people, a Rural Welfare Division has been established to devote special attention to the sociological aspects of the problem.

This brings me finally to the work of the Nutrition Division, to which I belong. Since the primary objective of the FAO is to raise nutritional levels throughout the world, it is essential that nutrition principles should be kept prominently before all the divisions and permeate FAO activities generally. The experts in other technical fields, such as agriculture, fisheries, forestry, and economics, must constantly be reminded to adapt their work to the primary needs of nutrition, not only to the need for sufficient food, but for food having a protein quality and other factors necessary to the health of man.

The FAO issues an annual report on the world food situation based on all available current information. These reports deal, not only with food production and supply, but also with the state of nutrition of the different populations. The Nutrition Division collects data for this purpose and collaborates with the Economics Division in preparing food balance sheets for each country, showing the number of calories and the single food factors available per capita of population. This needs intensive collaboration with the Division of Economics and Statistics.

The evaluation of energy values of different foodstuffs was studied by a committee in February, 1947, and a report, "Energy-yielding Components of Food and Computation of Calorie Values," was published. There are, of course, many facts known about these, but there is considerable difference of opinion between workers in North America and Europe about calculating the energy values of food, determining whether there is loss of values through cooking, etc. Even single food factors, especially carbohydrates in cereals and other foods, are not estimated along the same lines in all countries. The same is true in the case of the different vitamins for which common methods of estimation must be found. Calorie values of foodstuffs, especially of staple foods, are of considerable importance since the values employed may affect estimates of national food supplies and food requirements.

We are preparing international tables of food composition. Later, our tables will contain, in addition to the above-mentioned energy values, those of the accessory food factors also. It is not intended, however, to set up these tables on the basis of authority, but to collect existing data on a sound technical basis, to have an international basis for comparison and calculating.

A special problem is the methodology of assessment of nutritional status. Methods of determining health status must be ascertained from which the needs of populations can be judged. Moreover, dietary surveys must be prepared on a comparable basis for the same purpose.

A special phase of the work of the FAO is coöperation with the International Children's Emergency Fund of the United Nations. This organization supplies food of high nutritive value to children in war-devastated countries. Some four million children will receive aid through the ICEF, but much more help is needed. The Economic and Social Council of the United Nations recommended that the ICEF should not employ a technical staff, but should make full use of the technical services of the specialized agencies of the United Nations, such as the FAO and the WHO. In July, 1947, an expert committee was therefore convened by the FAO and WHO-Interim Commission to advise the ICEF. A number of specific recommendations were made to provide the Fund with technical advice and assistance. Two of our staff members, one of whom is stationed in Greece, work in close coöperation with the ICEF in Europe.

One of the most effective methods of improving nutritional status is school feeding. The FAO encourages, therefore, programs of school feeding in member countries, and we hope that an international report on this subject will be published.

A special problem is education in nutrition. There is no doubt that an astonishing world-wide ignorance of the basic facts of nutritional necessities exists. Many schools do not include nutritional education in their curricula. Even in the most advanced countries the housewife generally gets her information about food quality and food factors from newspaper advertisements. There is no doubt that such a situation opens the door to all kinds of misunderstanding. The situation becomes much worse in less advanced countries, especially where there are superstitions in food habits and primitive methods are still used because of lack of education in newer and easier methods. Nutritional education is a basic problem in countries with widespread malnutrition. We have worked out a voluminous report on rice-eating habits for the nutrition conference in Baguio in the Philippines and are proposing different ways to complete the diet of the rice-eater and to safeguard him from the methods of preparing his food that would ruin its nutritive value.

This leads to aspects of food technology. We are collecting

data on possibilities of using foods of high nutritional value which are at present not recognized as such mainly because people are not familiar with methods of preparing them in a palatable way. If we can find recipes that will make soybeans, food yeast, or even skimmed milk into preparations which will increase the demand for them, we will open great new resources for people in need.

To further the introduction of nutritional education in the schools as well as to inform the public and to influence the various governments through public opinion about good nutrition, we encourage the establishment of national nutrition organizations all over the world. Not every country is in such a fortunate position as the United States, which has institutions like the National Research Council with its Food and Nutrition Board, the Nutrition Foundation, and many other highly advanced research institutions in universities, agricultural colleges, and so on.

In its missions to various countries, such as Greece and Poland, the Nutrition Division of the FAO employed experts who were able to bring the findings of these commissions in line with nutrition principles. To spread a knowledge of nutrition, regional conferences are held, such as the Rice Conference in the Philippines, the Latin American Nutrition Conference, and the FAO Regional Conference held in Cairo in February, 1947.

Further regional work is under consideration by many of our member countries, and regional offices in which the Nutrition Division will coöperate are planned for Europe, the Near East, the Far East, and Latin America. The FAO is often asked for technical advice and assistance by less advanced parts of the world. The United States does not need outside help in studying and solving its nutrition problems, and an abundance of skilled personnel is available. But this is far from being the case in many other countries where they are most needed.

The FAO was created in 1945. Its constitution states as its objectives better levels of nutrition and standards of living, more efficient production and distribution of food and agricultural products, improved conditions for rural populations. But the goal of the FAO's immediate work is increased production of food and other essential products of farm, forest, and fishery, and the recommendation of allocations of scarce foods.

We are still building up this organization. One sees the walls of the building, one often cannot see all the finished details of the interior, and some of the rooms still cannot be used. Nevertheless, we are building with a long-term view that we may assure to future generations a better existence, but also, we are already working with the acute problems that are before us. If one should wait until agricultural development through large outside capital and an abundance of heavy equipment become available, perhaps little or nothing might be done. On the contrary, small projects, relatively inexpensive, can initiate in the immediate future a forward movement which may well make possible large and more ambitious undertakings later.

The FAO has vitality. This is proven by its continuous growth. There are now fifty-six member nations, which shows that the ideas which it represents appeal to the greater part of the world. In less developed countries there is certainly a deep determination to achieve economic development at a rapid rate. It is recognized as a most important principle of general economic development that agriculture must advance first, in order to produce a more adequate and more secure food supply. There is also a great need for economic coöperation to bring about the revival of production and trade and stable economic conditions in war-devastated countries. The member countries seem to realize that better diets for all, as well as fair and stable prices for producers and consumers of food products, should be the objectives of their policy. To build such an organization requires patience, good will, and the earnest help of experienced leaders.

We might close with the words spoken at the last FAO Conference in Geneva by Professor Friedrich T. Wahlen, of Switzerland, president of the Conference: "With its economic life severely disrupted by war the world urgently needs to re-establish itself on firm foundations. FAO is one of the agencies which must play a leading role in bringing about this process without which our entire civilization might well be overtaken by irreparable catastrophe."

And with the words of N. E. Dodd, chairman of the United States delegation to the FAO Conference in Geneva: "Progress today gives confidence in the hope that in FAO the world has an effective tool to bring about improved welfare for rural people and better food and health for all people."

Nursing for Health in Tomorrow's Family

RUTH W. HUBBARD

As I GAVE THOUGHT to tomorrow's family and the contribution of the nursing profession to that family's health, I asked myself six questions: Looking at today's family, can we foresee the family of tomorrow? Can we anticipate its needs, particularly in health? What may tomorrow's nurse be like? How will she work with families for their health? With whom will she work in behalf of these families? Is this pattern of service a design for all, or for some, and how can its values be secured in our American society?

Prophecy may be an exciting exercise. It is certainly a challenging and dangerous one, on the threshold of which I hesitate. Rather than risk a prophecy, I would like to base my idea of the future upon what now surrounds us in America. The pictures I shall suggest are one person's concept only and are presented as such. They grow out of living and working as a nurse of today.

Tomorrow's family—in the midst of the confusions and anxieties of today can we venture to describe the family of tomorrow? Not altogether accurately or clearly perhaps. Nevertheless, the experience of living in two generations leads me to suggest certain characteristics which, if true, will influence the opportunity and the service of tomorrow's nurse. In this country tomorrow's family may be smaller than yesterday's, may live more frequently in population centers, less often own its own home, will certainly do less basic preparation of its food while at the same time enjoying a wider variety than did its grandparents. The manual labor of homemaking will involve less strength and time from parents and children alike, but the decrease in the tasks in common for general family living may weaken some accepted strengths of family life.

The family as a whole will have more formal education and, in some instances, a wider range of adult educational opportunity. It appears that the custom of housing three-generation families under one roof may recur without a return to the more spacious living of the traditional farmhouse. Land, with its ownership, cultivation, and healing qualities, may less often be the family goal. A greater proportion of family members will move about the country and the world than formerly, and those who remain at home will be brought constantly in touch with the world by radio. The impact upon family life of outside influences, some good, some not good, cannot but be greater, and the resulting family awareness of the world will call for constant stabilizing effort through discriminating evaluation and judgment.

The family's new freedom of movement will bring also a corresponding sense of responsibility for the welfare of peoples no longer totally strange or remote. It may be less easy to develop enduring purposefulness and serenity. Certainly, organized society has made great progress in creating community resources to foster family well-being, while the worker in every field has won greater freedom through shorter working hours and heavier pay envelopes.

Those families of tomorrow who are already laying their foundations give us great courage and often inspiration. Interrupted, as many of them were by a world war, they are nevertheless purposeful, adaptable, resourceful, ready for fun, but intent on reaching an established objective in the family and abroad. They show attributes of a pioneer spirit and they are not readily fooled. Those who seek to be of service to them must, to use the slang expression, "be good." They think, they work, and they are not easily discouraged. But subject as they are to the influences of a world that flounders and a society that is uncertain, they too will need help often and of many kinds. May the community services of tomorrow be ready. No longer will agencies through their staffs do things *to* people. Services may be rendered *for* people, but problems will be solved *with* people, and coöperative effort in its truest sense will emerge, not easily or smoothly, but, I believe, surely.

This family of tomorrow will certainly have health needs. Environmental sanitation and disease control have altered the type of need in two generations. Yet experience teaches that vigilance alone insures safety. Unused knowledge or ignorance in the presence of knowledge is no safeguard. The acute illnesses of childhood have diminished, child bearing and rearing have become less hazardous, yet other unsolved problems press forward in the prevention and control of illness. Can we, then, hope to direct a successful campaign toward healthful living with illness still so common a lot of mankind?

The answer is certainly yes, for the family outlook toward illness and health is changing. There is a new, challenging attitude that does not accept illness as inevitable nor handicap as insurmountable. The family of tomorrow will want to enjoy good health and use to the full its several individual resources. These resources, physical, emotional, intellectual, economic, may not be perfect, but the family will not hide its talents in a napkin for safekeeping. It will need to know how to nourish healthy bodies, as well as to bear them; how to budget income, as well as to earn it; how to adjust to the restrictions of long-term illness smoothly, as well as to meet the emergencies of accident and acute illness. Learning to understand and use the strengths of family life while not giving way to its strains may not come easily, but now the community offers tested help in mental hygiene.

Tomorrow's nurse—can we see her clearly?

Nursing as a profession is about seventy-five years old in this country. It has experienced the natural struggles of an evolving group and has emerged with a recognized body of knowledge; this period has been one of formal preparation which involves the mastery of specific scientific knowledge and skills through clinical experience; the years have brought a widening range of acceptable opportunities for service; and the profession has been embraced by a rapidly growing group of women (and some men) as a way of life.

Furthermore, nursing has developed a quality which to me has great meaning. It is the welcome which patients and colleagues have afforded to this new professional worker. I do not minimize the importance of the other characteristics of a profession, but I believe that our greatest justification for further effort toward usefulness lies in the fact that the pioneers proved themselves helpful in a manner readily accepted by the American family, physician, health officer, social worker, and community worker.

In the past century the whole concept of the contribution of a nurse has changed. In the beginning she was principally occupied with alleviating the difficulties of illness and was seldom employed in preventing the occurrence of illness. But medicine's breathtaking advance in disease prevention during the last fifty years enables all workers in the field of health and welfare to set new and, we believe, attainable goals in national health.

This change, so welcome, but as yet so far from realization, has developed the nurse of today whose interest, preparation, and skills enable her to accept these responsibilities and to function accordingly. Tomorrow's nurse will continue to be concerned with the care of those who are ill. But, like the nurse of today, she will have as great, if not greater concern for the maintenance and promotion of health. This health is not merely the absence of disease, but a far more positive state of well-being which frees the individual to expend all his gifts, interests, and strength on the fullest possible attainment of his personal contribution to the society in which he lives, and his receipt, in turn, of satisfactions therefrom. Tomorrow's nurse may more nearly see the realization of this concept.

A group of younger nurses who assisted in making a study of nursing schools have described the nurse in a manner helpful for our consideration at this point:

It is the opinion of this group that in the latter half of the 20th Century, the professional nurse will be one who recognizes and understands fundamental needs of a person, sick or well, and who knows how these needs can best be met. She will possess a body of scientific nursing knowledge which is based upon and keeps pace with general scientific advancement, and she will be able to apply this knowledge in meeting the nursing needs of a person and community. She must possess that kind of discriminative judgment which will enable her to recognize those activities which fall within the area of professional nursing and those activities which have been identified within the fields of other professional or non-professional groups.

She must be able to exert leadership in at least four different ways: (1) in making her unique contribution to the preventive and remedial aspects of illness; (2) in improving those nursing skills already in existence and developing new nursing skills; (3) in teaching and supervising other nurses and auxiliary workers; (4) in coöperating with other professions in planning for positive health on community, state, national and international levels.[1]

How can this nurse of tomorrow work with her families? First, I must tell you where I think she will work. Nurses have penetrated into almost all the places where people live and work, and I believe that this penetration will be completed. But I think that the nurse will render her major service for health to families in their homes, for it is in the home that the family lives and that the life of the family takes its form.

The person who hopes to help a family to healthful living must be familiar with, and understanding of, the family individually and collectively. She must be able to meet each family on its own ground and respond to the needs that its members can express as well as to those they exhibit. The nurse (and I am speaking here of the community nurse) who is a frequent visitor to the home, and who, in consequence, sees the family in crisis and in calm, has the richest opportunity to observe the family's way of life. If she is a skilled and understanding observer, she can make wise use of these observations in her own service to the family and in her relationship to others who are either active in, or are needed for, providing assistance for the family. As a countryman learns to evaluate the weather signs in his neighborhood by living there for more than a holiday, so the nurse who comes re-

[1] "Nursing in the Second Half of the 20th Century," in Esther Lucile Brown, *The Professional Nurse of the Future* (New York: Russell Sage Foundation, 1948), p. 73.

peatedly into the home learns to judge what she finds by relating it to a succession of earlier visits.

How? That is the real question. Seven ways suggest themselves: the skill of the nurse in discovering the family's own sense of need for help in problems of health; her ability to recognize and accept the family's readiness to accept help as it presents itself (and this may not always be what she feels to be of first importance); basic knowledge so much a part of her that she can adapt it freely to each individual family; ingenuity, skill, and patience in timing advice and suggestion; adequate knowledge of available health and medical resources and the way in which they can be used; a fundamental appreciation of her professional function as one member of a team which enables her to work with and through the other healing arts professions in behalf of her family; and a freedom from judgment, coupled with perseverance, that insures her willingness to try again. I have covered all but the sense of humor; it is certainly indicated and it will be there.

I am not deliberately sidestepping a recital of method. Instead, I have tried to indicate an individual concept of the families of tomorrow and the nurse who may work with them. Her method will vary with each family, although her goal will not change. A number of years ago the public health nurse was honored by being called "the enabling clause of public health legislation." If she is truly an "enabling clause," she is definitely two things. she is always a part of a larger group working for the same ends, and she is able to adapt the form of her service to the particular family in question. As a member of the health team she has the unique function of interpreting its message to her family so that they can use it while she helps them to marshal their resources (physical, emotional, mental, social, economic) as well as those of the community in behalf of the problem to be solved, taking the time to develop the confidence which is based on proven service and assisting in the development of the family's self-dependence.

This leads me to the fifth question: With whom does the nurse work in behalf of her families? I have suggested that I see her as a member of a team. This concept is decidedly an emerging one in our century, but lest it appear that the nurse of tomorrow will attempt to spread herself too broadly and to be all things to all people, let me emphasize my belief that she is but one member of a growing group in our society which works in behalf of family health. The family, the physician always, the social worker, the schoolteacher, and the minister often, are recognized members of this team. Others are called in consultation, and as our knowledge increases still more members may appear. To work together to advance general community health and welfare is our accepted American procedure. To do so in behalf of individual families is a growing concept and one on which rests to a large extent, I believe, our hope for successful outcome.

The rapid advance along the frontiers of knowledge in the field of community health and welfare has resulted in needed extensive specialization. But the well-being of the individual patient and his family in diagnosis, treatment, and the maintenance of health depends upon the establishment of continuous, integrated assistance and guidance. This is best assured by teamwork in the finest meaning of the word. The point is already accepted in practice. It flourishes, where it is appreciated, even with limited staffs and crowded schedules as one of the best timesavers and assurances of successful work.

Finally, the sixth question: Is nursing for health in the family a pattern for all, and if so how can it be secured for the American family? The Community Service Society has developed an outstanding example of the very service we have been discussing. It has done so carefully, painstakingly, with great vision. To determine sound procedure and to insure a fair trial, it has used the freedom of a voluntary agency to set its experiment and to carry it out scientifically in a controlled situation. The results speak for themselves in the report of a century of war on poverty and disease as well as on environmental health and social hazards. Can the American families of tomorrow, from the Atlantic to the Pacific, from the Great Lakes to the Gulf, anticipate a similar service? This is, perhaps, the ultimate test. It involves such queries as: Can all families use such a service profitably? Do other problems call more imperatively for solution? Can all communities support the workers? Can nursing education prepare the nurses? Can schools of nursing secure the quality and number of potential workers needed? These questions are not easily answered even in a country of resources like the United States.

In the present period of postwar self-examination we are confronted by an ever mounting list of urgent situations that call upon united community action for their solution. Yet as never before in the world's history mankind is conscious of the importance of the well-being of each person to the well-being of society. In the last 100 years four major wars have shaken the country, no less than five economic depressions have paralyzed human courage and energies. In the same period, medical sciences have made breath-taking strides, and in this present century alone the expected span of life has increased fifteen years. The Community Service Society has made the vision of a healthy, full life a reality for a small number of families who are surrounded by millions of families for whom the goal is only a dream. The discovery of a way, the charting of a course, are gifts of rare price. The extension of the benefits to all our countrymen, to all the world, in fact, is the challenge before us now.

Until recently, a large measure of the nursing practice in this country was directed toward the care and recovery of the sick. Only within the last quarter century has any sizable number of nurses practiced principally for the promotion of health and the prevention of disease. The majority of families still seek health assistance from physician, dentist, and nurse on the basis of its recognized absence. Dr. C. E. A. Winslow reminds us that "the disease of poverty affects a proportion not far from one-third of our population." [2]

Dr. Louis I. Dublin points out that "careful forecasts indicate that by 1960 almost one-third of our population will be 45 years of age and over," and that,

[some] 70% of our invalids, that is persons permanently disabled, are at ages 45 or higher. The pattern of disease incidence, like mortality, has shifted to feature the conditions of the older ages. Thus, in the countrywide Metropolitan nursing experience for policyholders in

[2] C. E. A. Winslow, "Poverty and Disease," *American Journal of Public Health*, XXXVIII (January, 1948), 173–84.

1925 nearly 50% of the cases were nursed for the acute and communicable conditions, most of which occur in early life, and only about 5% were for the chronic diseases, conditions typical of old age; in 1945, on the other hand, the two figures were 14% and 28% respectively. A complete reversal in emphasis has taken place.[3]

While no accurate figures are available on the proportion of persons ill at home who require nursing care, Dr. Dublin makes the suggestion that one nurse to every 5,000 of population (about 28,000 nurses) is needed for this service. Dr. Parran has said that 60,000 public health nurses are needed immediately for all public health nursing services in the country as a whole.

These observations, coupled with extensive experience in a voluntary public health nursing association whose service is based on bedside care, lead me to take a middle-of-the-road position. The public health nurse of tomorrow will have a distinct nursing contribution to make to the health of tomorrow's family; she may make this best if her services include the care of the sick.

Here I come to the heart of my message. The family of tomorrow that I have attempted to envision will have goals in health which we, as members of the health team, can help them to achieve. I have ventured to suggest that our American families are already making such demands of us and are using the help that the team, functioning imperfectly as yet, now offers. Tomorrow they will make even better use of us if we are ready.

Today and tomorrow the nurse who nurses for health in a family nurses sickness also. Almost every family has at some time an illness situation which it must meet. The nurse who is concerned with the well-being of her family is present at such times. One of her great strengths is the continuity of her service. In sickness and in health her service is valued. In many families today—and tomorrow—health and sickness occur simultaneously. The pattern may be successive or concurrent. The nurse who lives up to the highest aspects of her calling functions helpfully in both, and, in my belief, more effectively if she is free to do just

[3] Louis I. Dublin, "Problems of an Aging Population: Setting the Stage," *American Journal of Public Health*, XXXVII (February, 1947), 152–62.

that. All the trends toward generalization in individual service and unification in the organized public health services lead me to this answer.

If society can equip the nurse to render health and curative services alike to her families, she will most truly "nurse for health." Life does not divide us as individuals or families into watertight compartments of sickness and health. Each one of us and every family experiences both. To nurse in sickness is to nurse a patient with a disease. To nurse for family health is to nurse a family for its health. These are not arbitrary, stereotyped services but, as is well appreciated, highly individualized adaptations of established knowledges and skills.

Twenty-five years ago in a tiny Scottish seaside town a distinguished cardiologist unwittingly gave me this ideal. Because it had become his goal in medicine, he had withdrawn from a great London practice to live with, study, observe, and practice among, a small group of people. In this way only, he said, could he come to know his patients intimately enough to foster their health, to anticipate the course of disease in them, to control and minimize its effects, and to advise them wisely in living their own lives in health and illness. In a generation of such service Sir James Mackenzie gave invaluable assistance to his patients, to research, and to practicing physicians throughout the world.

If society can provide for tomorrow the public health nursing service we have endeavored to suggest here in quantity sufficient to secure continuous as well as skillful understanding nurse-and-family relationship, then I truly believe that the ideal pattern of service can be woven creatively into the design of our American family health.

Achieving Family Health through Modern Education

ERNEST OSBORNE

THERE IS A TENDENCY in all professional fields to develop attitudes and practices which become sacrosanct. The majority of the members of any given profession are likely to accept such attitudes and practices as rooted in some universal absolute. Criticisms or even suggestions from laymen and from workers in allied professions are discounted because those who make them are not bona fide members of the fraternity. Out of such protective, defensive attitudes comes sterility.

It is heartening, then, when the social work profession turns to workers in other fields and asks them to think together, to pool their varied experiences, and to move forward toward at least the beginnings of an effective integration of the experience and wisdom which severally they have developed. Any full-blown development of this trend will not come easily, though there are evidences of it in a number of professional groups. There will be disappointments, too, at some of the results. It is no easy thing for us to coöperate. Even those anxious for such cross-fertilization and integration of practice in the service professions will find the path rough at times.

An educator who attempts to discuss the role of modern education in achieving health is susceptible to several weaknesses. He may dwell on trick motivations, on "gimmicks," or on "cute" approaches. Far too often attempts have been made to develop health programs through superficial and specious methods. He may find it comfortable to make a show of being erudite, of developing an involved analysis of the laws of learning and of their

Family Health through Education

application to health education. He may, too, make that most common mistake of considering "education" as synonymous with "schooling."

In an attempt to avoid these pitfalls, it seems best to select several developing educational concepts that are generally accepted in modern education although they may not be widely practiced:

1. The individual is an integral part of all his experiences and cannot be intelligently considered apart from them; of these experiences, his relationships with his family are most significant.

Acceptance of this concept by educators has led to efforts to develop closer home-school relationships, among other things. It is more and more clearly recognized that behavior difficulties as shown in school and elsewhere are closely tied to interpersonal relationships within the family. A simple and convincing example is found in certain compulsive drives for attention which show themselves in several ways. The youngster may constantly cling to the teacher, he may be unusually noisy in the classroom, or he may show the "chip-on-the-shoulder" attitude toward his classmates. This type of symptomatic behavior is almost invariably associated with family-centered factors, such as the arrival of a new child, favoritism shown toward a sibling, or the use of invidious comparison.

We know, too, that basic social attitudes are derived out of home experiences. Consideration on the part of the child for the welfare of companions, for example, is usually a reflection, not only of expressed attitudes of parents, but of the ways in which these parents show consideration for their children. It has often been said that the roots of prejudice are in the home. The converse is naturally also true; understanding and acceptant attitudes and practices toward those who differ racially, religiously, or economically are most effectively determined, not in social studies classes in the school nor even in the ethical and religious teachings of Sunday school, but out of the pervasive security of understanding and loving parents whose every action attests their concern for persons. Whether or not there is talk of the brotherhood of man, the value of individual personality, or the importance of equality and justice, day-by-day living of these ideals roots them deep in the growing child.

How, then, will such a concept apply to the field of health? Among the practices to be avoided is one once common in health education—the use of the child as a kind of health missionary sent out from the school to convert his parents' and the family's health habits. With the best intentions in the world, those who use such a procedure are as likely to arouse friction and antagonism among family members as they are to succeed in eliminating the use of a family drinking glass or in securing the brushing of teeth after every meal. It would seem far more important that good parent-child relationships be maintained than that some picayune victories on the health front be gained.

Indeed, if we accept the implications of the concept, we will recognize that a warm, acceptant relationship among the members of the family is a primary health objective. More and more clearly we are seeing the unhealthy effects of anxiety engendered in both child and parent by nagging, withdrawal of affection, or other negatively charged attempts to secure conformity to a relatively unimportant series of concrete behaviors that supposedly mark the "well-brought-up" child. It is interesting to note, too, how frequently the child takes advantage of parental anxiety to control the family. The eating situation provides one of the most common examples. When mother, father, or grandmother begin to fear that Junior is not eating enough and develop a series of futile, though ingenious, appeals to get him to eat, it is clear who is "boss." The child rightly judges how important his eating is to his family and uses this information as a whip to make the family toe the mark and to dance attendance on him.

Recognition of the significance of such family interaction will also lead us to try to develop deeper understanding of the ways in which parental attitudes bring about certain functional concepts toward health and illness on the part of children. In a number of ways, often unrecognized, parents may, by their attitudes and behavior, build into children dynamic feelings toward health and illness.

An excessive concern with cleanliness is likely to develop a kind of "bacteria phobia" which has both personal and social disadvantages. There are, of course, a number of possible Freudian implications involved, such as guilt rising out of earlier feelings of rejection leading to frantic overconcern with protective measures against possible disease. Whatever the cause, the result is far too often an individual who continues to be obsessed with cleanliness.

Some parents may think of illness as something about which to be ashamed. Children are scolded for their carelessness in becoming ill. Such an attitude, though avoiding the pitfalls of overconcern, may bring about a refusal to care for oneself when a cold is developing or the ignoring of symptoms which should warn of an onset of illness. If parents have used the shame motive strongly and consistently, then the sense of guilt about being ill will get in the way of an intelligent attitude toward medical treatment and even toward protective methods.

More common than either of these is the use of illness as an escape from situations that are hard to face. In varying degrees this is almost universal. Monday morning stomach-aches of the child who is not getting along too well in school, vague physical symptoms in a graduate student who is facing a stiff examination at the end of the term, the larger number of migraine headaches, and many similar physical manifestations are familiar to us all. Here again, the genesis of such reactions can usually be traced to parental failure to help the youngster, who naturally begins to make use of such methods to avoid unpleasant situations, face his problems realistically. It is also true, of course, that children whose mother or father makes use of illness to avoid responsibility or to justify otherwise unjustifiable behavior tend to follow similar behavior patterns.

2. A sound educational process starts with the individual where he is and is rooted in his needs, his interests, and even his prejudices.

In spite of all the evidence to the contrary most people like to assume that man is essentially a logical creature and that once presented with the facts of a situation, it is only willfulness that keeps him from acting on these facts. This has been largely true of health education. In practice, we have said again and again, "Here are the facts as to the way in which you should care for yourself. They are based on scientific evidence. Of course, you will want to follow them." The fact is that a variety of motivations causes individuals to do the things which are "good for them," but cool reason and clear logic come far down on the list. What are the realities? The following indicate a few of the more dynamic ones:

a) Children and youth want to consider themselves "grown-up" and will assume the practices and attitudes which their observation of adult behavior leads them to believe are characteristically "grown-up" activities.

Far too often, smoking, drinking, and staying up late are thought of as being adult prerogatives and, consequently, badges of maturity. No matter that it is pointed out that these are not "good" for the younger generation, they still are symbolic of being "grown-up." The educational problem involved here is not a simple one. Children must be helped to accept the fact that certain activities are acceptable for adults but not desirable for younger persons. This may not be too easy, however, and often will constitute a point on which complete acceptance is difficult.

The goal of parents, teachers, and other adult leaders should be one of interpreting as effectively as possible desirable practices as being the "grown-up" ones. The youngster may be led to pattern his practices on those of the college athlete who follows training-table regulations or of the motion picture actress who must get plenty of rest if she is to remain in top form. Unfortunately, one cannot always count on consistent behavior on the part of those who are used as examples. In spite of the difficulties involved, a candid and honest approach to discrepancies must be maintained, or any value in the use of an adult example is likely to be negated.

b) Young persons as well as adults often hold immediate and passing values in higher esteem than they do long-term and continuing goals.

The force of the immediate, the lack of ability to accept the

Family Health through Education

long-term goal, is another perplexing phenomenon in the whole process of an intelligent approach to the guidance of youth. There are many interesting examples. One which is relatively common should be sufficient to illustrate the strength of the here and now in motivating behavior.

To the sixteen-year-old star basketball player, the current acclaim for his ability is likely to weigh more heavily than the doctor's statement that continued playing may permanently impair his heart. To the parent, teacher, or adult friend of the family, such an attitude seems completely foolish, and they rarely show any sympathy with it. Unless, however, some comparable way of gaining social approval from their peers can be found, most adolescents will find it very difficult to be "sensible." In such instances every effort should be made to substitute some positive and approval-gaining activity for the usual nagging or exhortation to use one's common sense.

Likewise, the personal need to appear vigorous and healthy to one's peers—to be able to keep up—will be felt to be more important than the individual need for more rest and care than the average person requires. Persons, whether adults or adolescents, who because of heart, lung, or other physical condition should not overtax themselves must be helped, where this is at all possible, to find a way of life that does not make them conspicuously different from their fellows.

c) "Unworthy" motives may be more determinative of behavior than appeals to the "higher self."

Here again one sees that reason, "good sense," and other practical factors are rarely as potent in affecting behavior as are self-centered concerns. So, for instance, if a young mother who is not completely prepared emotionally for the responsibilities of parenthood is helped to realize that the infant thus treated will be less fussy and troublesome, she may be more effectively motivated to keep her baby clean and dry than if the emphasis were put on her love for the child or her pride in being a good mother.

The whole emphasis in our culture on personal attractiveness, though often carried to a nauseating extreme by advertisers, may likewise be a much more realistic motivation than an appeal which more soberly calls for care of one's health so that the body may function at its highest potential.

Another point seems to be worth mentioning here. Our deadly serious concern with health practices sometimes leads us to emphasize an unswerving and rigid adherence to what is known to be desirable. It would seem that to "let down" a bit now and then has certain psychological advantages. A dietary "binge" or an occasional late bedtime has a certain release value and makes it easier for child or youth generally to adopt the good health habits that we advise for him.

It is not always easy to see what is implied if we accept this concept of starting with the learner where he is. There will have to be a bit of trial and error. Nevertheless, the principle is sound and will result in far better responses from the learners than the attitude which insists on conformity to practices which they do not understand and fully accept.

3. *The active participation of the individuals concerned in the development of any program is an essential part of its success.*

With varying degrees of thoroughness, modern education attempts to develop active participation of the learner in the educational process. By and large, today's youngsters learn more effectively than did most of their parents to take responsibility, to make intelligent choices, to coöperate effectively with others in the many aspects of the modern school's activities. In what ways is it feasible to apply this principle of the value of participation to the field of health?

To begin with, we must recognize one phenomenon that would seem to run counter to the idea that it is desirable to participate actively in any venture of which one is a part. Over and over again, one finds that many people want precise, definite formulas or prescriptions by which to govern their actions. Parents want specific directions as to what to do when their children refuse to obey, pinch the cat, or otherwise engage in reprehensible activities. Many teachers like to have step-by-step curricula planned for them so that few choices will have to be made. And so it is with individuals from almost any group. Out of our childhood experiences in home, school, and community we have

Family Health through Education

learned—too many of us—to be more comfortable when others make the decisions. Consciously or unconsciously, we strive to maintain this painless state of affairs.

To some workers in every field, this sort of dependence on a leader, an expert, seems to be a desirable state of affairs. They enjoy the complete dependence of their children, their students, the members of their congregation, or their patients. But such a relationship, satisfying as it may seem at times, has within it at least three grave weaknesses.

First, the dependents may become a nuisance. Witness the young mother who calls the doctor whenever her child shows the slightest symptom of illness rather than learning through experience when she can safely rely upon her own judgment.

Secondly, the dependents are not likely to be discriminating. The very attitude that permits them unquestioningly to accept the expert's word means that they may as likely follow demagogues or quacks or become equally uncritical devotees of some health cult.

Less dramatic than these two weaknesses but more important is a third factor. Because of their intimate knowledge of particular children, parents in the home, teachers in the classroom, any adult living closely with children or youth day by day, are potentially capable of detecting signs of illness that even a well-trained doctor or nurse might overlook. School health authorities recognize this and encourage classroom teachers to look for the symptoms of incipient illness that may be detected during the day's activities but are not apparent during an examination in the school health office. One illustration will indicate ways in which alert parents may learn to know their child's reactions in such a way as to detect the onset of illness. Whenever Douglas, who was eight years of age, showed unusual courtesy toward all about him and was outstandingly gracious, his mother was sure that he was coming down with a fever. This unusual reaction had been noted through a period of years and naturally would be one which a doctor could hardly be expected to understand had he not had the same close contacts with the boy. Many similar idiosyncrasies can be found among youngsters. Every effort should be made to encourage parents to become aware of them and thus play one of their significant roles in maintaining and promoting the health of members of the family.

a) One guide to the effectiveness of any program or relationship is the degree to which it leaves individuals better able to meet situations independently, to know when expert help is needed but to use their own good judgment increasingly in deciding when home care is all that is needed.

Recent discussion with a public health nurse high-lighted for me an educational procedure which seems very promising, one that is used too seldom in any sort of education. When she goes into a home she "thinks out loud" with the parent, first to help her face the facts in the situation, and second to help develop the ability of her patient to carry through more independently in similar situations. Let us imagine that the nurse has been called in to see a frightened young mother of a first baby because the mother reports that the baby has diarrhea. The nurse is busy, and it would take only a short time to observe that the healthy, contented baby has no fever and to find out that the child is taking feedings well and sleeping well. However, she does not dismiss the mother's fears lightly until she has reviewed the whole situation with her. This involves "thinking out loud" about what may have caused the bowel movements to increase and to be loose. If the baby is breast fed, was extra sugar put in; or was an oily vitamin preparation recently added to the child's diet, etc., etc.? The diapers are examined, and the mother is helped to see that the stool is not so different from what it has been and told what to look for in case a real diarrhea develops. A review of the symptoms that would indicate the necessity for a doctor's care and of what to do if such a situation should arise is part of the education here, too. This will all take more time, but the nurse's interest and concern will reassure the mother, she will be less frightened, and she will learn more readily the facts that the nurse is teaching. It seems obvious that in another such experience, she will be better prepared to meet the situation without panic and with intelligent judgment.

The sense of security which such an approach is likely to de-

Family Health through Education

velop is most desirable. In health education programs in our schools this Socratic approach—use of questions—sharing in the exploration of the realities of health is likely to be far more effective than subject matter that is set out to be learned.

b) Development of a skeptical or critical attitude is one of the important emphases in modern education.

Children are guided to ask constantly: "What is the evidence for this statement?" "Are the facts behind this conclusion sound ones?" "Is the interpretation presented, one based on the facts?" In the area of health practice, it is surely just as important to develop this questioning attitude as in any other field. In schools where youngsters are encouraged to question advertising related to health, where they are helped to ferret out "quack" ideas about health, where they learn to suspend judgment regarding practices about which the experts disagree, one sees the beginnings of the kind of mature judgment we need in effectively functioning citizens of a democracy. Even intelligent adults have many twisted ideas concerning health practices and medical care. There is much to be done.

c) The development of this kind of active participation in the learning process can be forwarded effectively through the organization of a representative health and safety council.

Through the health and safety council, children of all ages, with the counsel of adults, can study the particular health and safety hazards existing in their school, canvass the opinions of their fellow students, consult experts on specific problems, and in all sorts of ways concern themselves with bringing about better conditions in the school, in the home, and even in the community. We in America have not provided enough significant opportunities for children and youth to participate in the improvement of school, home, and community practices. As junior citizens in a democracy they should be provided with such opportunities.

In a few communities, I understand, lay participation in the modification of clinic procedures has been developed. Who is better equipped to play a part in analyzing organized health services and in bringing about needed changes than the consumer himself? To be sure, there are technical limitations, but so far as the way in which people respond to services provided, so far as suggestions for added service, and so far as ideas for reaching and serving more people are concerned, the layman has much to contribute.

At home, too, through family councils, all the members of the family should share in the making of decisions which, among other things, deal with health practices. A family discussion of the time at which it is reasonable to expect the younger members of the family to return from evening social engagements, a discussion concerning the need for regular medical and dental check-ups or in regard to any of a dozen family matters directly or indirectly concerned with health, will result in wiser and more acceptable plans and decisions than those made by parents only.

There are still many things left unsaid. I have an uneasy feeling that some of them may be more important than those to which I have given some attention. But I believe there can be little argument as to the major concepts I have tried to develop. We know that the individual is a part of all his experiences and his relationships. We are agreed that effective education starts with the learner where he is. We are convinced that active participation in the learning is more effective than passive absorption of verbalized concepts. But we are all falling short of doing much that is realistic about this knowledge, these agreements, or these convictions.

We need much more thinking and planning together, we can learn much from one another. We must join forces, break down the professional protective walls that keep us from working harmoniously and effectively together.

Professional Interplay for Family Health

HUGH R. LEAVELL, M.D., DR.P.H.

As WE DISCUSS PROFESSIONAL INTERPLAY for family health, let us think of ourselves as exploring ways to develop a championship team in the big game of health promotion for the families of our communities. Many professions furnish team members, and so diverse are the family's health needs that all must play in the game to supply the special techniques each can contribute. Some play in the line, doing unspectacular but still very necessary jobs. Others, in the back field, carry the ball, throwing forward passes now and again to the ends. Only occasionally may we hope to find a single back equally capable of punting, passing, and running the ball. Usually, each team member may be counted upon merely for his own special skill.

We must clarify the rules of the game at the outset by staking out the territory to be included in our discussion. The word "health" we shall use in its broad sense as it is used in the World Health Organization constitution: "a state of complete physical, mental and social well-being and not merely the absence of disease and infirmity."[1] We must, as does the American Medical Association, include medical care of the sick as part of a comprehensive health program.[2] We recognize that in the modern sense, health activities have four essential phases: promotion of health; prevention of ill health; cure or alleviation of disease and injury;

[1] "Constitution of the World Health Organization," *Public Health Reports*, LXI (August 30, 1946), 1268–79.
[2] "The Ten Point National Health Program of the American Medical Association," *Journal of the American Medical Association*, CXXXVI (January 24, 1948), 261–66.

and rehabilitation of the disabled.[3] In speaking of a "profession," we refer, according to *Webster's New International Dictionary*, to "a calling in which one professes to have acquired some special skill used by way of either instructing, guiding or advising others or of serving them in some art." An "interplay" is defined as "mutual action or influence." The word "family" is used in the sense in which it is used in the Peckham Experiment, as nature's building unit in the biological world, a "mated pair either with or as yet without children." In speaking, then, of "professional interplay for family health," we are approaching our subject rather broadly.

As practically every known profession has some stake in promoting family health, there would be little profit in attempting to draw up an inclusive list. Educators, social workers, the ministry, and all branches of medicine and public health would have special prominence in such an enumeration. If we keep in mind the four phases of health activity referred to previously, especially is it apparent that our undertaking is really quite amazingly complex. There is little wonder the average family is confused by the maze of specialists in this or that field who must be consulted about one phase or another of the family's health. Fortunately, health interests the general public immensely; otherwise, the average family surely would not have sufficient energy and enthusiasm to see the complicated job through.

Let us put ourselves in the position of the coach of our family health team. We must do everything possible to make sure that the team members have as complete knowledge as possible of the health needs and problems of the family. They must know the requirements in the physical, psychological, and environmental spheres in so far as present information permits. There must be some background of historical information about family development and understanding of changes taking place under the impact of socio-economic forces active in the world today. Training in professional schools can meet only partially this need for

[3] Henry Gluckman, chairman, "Report of the National Health Services Commission on the Provision of an Organized National Health Service for All Sections of the People of the Union of South Africa 1942–1944" (Pretoria: Government Printer, 1944), pp. 8–10.

basic knowledge. Our team members must continue the learning process throughout their entire professional lives. As research methods of the social sciences develop more completely, we may expect new information of inestimable value to them. Kinsey, in his interesting book, warns us against fear that research will not have popular support: "Even the scientist seems to have underestimated the faith of the man in the street in the scientific method, his respect for the results of scientific research, and his confidence that his own life and the whole of the social organization will ultimately benefit from the accumulation of scientifically established data." [4]

Each team member must clearly understand his own assignment in the promotion of family health. In addition, he needs to know what his teammates can contribute with their varying skills. Here, we must demand of the professional schools a much better job than most of them have done in the past. In some schools there are already admirable arrangements for presenting the picture of a health service which has a real unity. Students privileged to observe the example of unification found in the Community Service Society with its caseworkers and public health personnel coöperating so intimately are much more fortunate than those who cannot see such an excellent service in actual operation. Nevertheless, opportunities exist wherever there are training facilities worthy of approval by national certifying bodies. In Pittsburgh, medical students and social workers in training join in classes where social, economic, and medical problems are discussed by the case study method. In schools of medicine, dentistry, nursing, and public health, socio-economic case studies involving home visits and reasonably prolonged follow-up by the students must become the rule rather than the exception. In such studies, students should gain clear insight into the methods and contributions of social workers, educators, ministers, and other groups which have assisted in solving the family problem, or could assist had they been called upon. Donald Bertrand Tresidder, President of Stanford University, stressed

---

[4] A. C. Kinsey, W. B. Pomeroy, and C. E. Martin, *Sexual Behavior in the Human Male* (Philadelphia: Saunders, 1948), p. 4.

the importance of such training recently in saying, "I have the strongest conviction that the first aim of medical education, aside from the development of professional competence, should be to give the student a clear understanding that from first to last, he will have a great concern with social problems. . . . the doctor, of all people, will require social skills and insight into social problems of the highest order." [5]

The practice of having theological students serve an "internship" in hospitals is excellent. It gives them an opportunity to see the complexity of hospital organization and how they best can fit themselves into hospital life to make their contribution most effective. These students and the hospital chaplains can show medical personnel and social workers the value of the religious element in promoting family health. They may also have suggestions useful for hospital administrators as to how their institutions might be run for greater benefit of the patients. Minister-psychiatrist teams are opening up great untilled areas of coöperative activity with boundless possibilities. One sometimes wonders whether social workers have grasped fully the dynamic possibilities of incorporating religious therapy more completely into their schemes of treatment.

In our plans for furthering professional interplay for family health, it is likely that we may have to go back beyond the training offered by professional schools and revise their admission policies. Applicants for medical schools must meet certain basic natural science requirements for admission. These are, of course, essential for understanding the medical curriculum. Recently, however, some voices in the wilderness have cried for increased emphasis on broader background training in social sciences and humanities. Since many medical schools have recruited their students selectively, practically to exclude those with consuming interest in coöperative social activity, why should we be surprised at having a generation of doctors who are more concerned with scientific medicine than with the patient? There is reason to believe that social workers would, on the other hand, profit

[5] D. B. Tresidder, "The Aims and Purposes of Medical Education," *Journal of the Association of American Medical Colleges*, XXIII (January, 1948), 8–17.

by more natural science in their preprofessional training. The broader our backgrounds, the easier it is going to be for all of us to work together.

We would be shortsighted if we were to place complete dependence on colleges and professional schools in developing this knowledge of what the other groups are doing. Staff conferences and in-service training must be used to further the process. It is commendable for members of each profession to feel that their own contribution is essential or even more important than that of any other group. On the other hand, it is decidedly wrong to minimize the work of other professions and even worse to have little or no knowledge of it. "The health team cannot be a closed circle of in-facing initiates with backs to the outside world; rather, it must be an open circle ready to welcome new workers and able to expand as new areas of useful coöperation are discovered." [6]

We must recognize and take into account certain very definite limitations on professional interplay. There are elements of trade unionism which have a restrictive influence. Jurisdictional disputes and boycotts have occurred even in the professions under discussion. Jealousy is by no means unheard of, and there is a nearsightedness with which the eye specialists cannot deal. Scientists profit somewhat by a sort of shorthand in their speech, but the incomprehensible jargon and gobbledegook which too often develop, erect almost impenetrable barriers to effective coöperation from other groups. The more fully a common sort of basic English can be used, the easier it is going to be for us all to work together.

Terrific personnel shortages restrict effective planning for teamwork in many fields today. Psychiatrists and nurses are in such short supply that it is nearly impossible to set up balanced community programs involving these professional groups. Other shortages are nearly as obvious, notably in the teaching profession. Adequate recruitment for future needs must not be based upon attractive salaries alone if we are to have the really best

[6] Paul E. Johnson, "Religious Psychology and Health," *Mental Hygiene*, XXXI (October, 1947), 555–66.

material for our future program. Means must be found to present the glamour of these healing professions in the true light that is so amply justified. Many of us seem a little ashamed to be engaged in a life of service and may even lose sight of the enormous satisfactions to be derived from such dedication. While this type of service will not clothe and feed one's family, it is, nevertheless, a factor to be reckoned with in presenting the attractions of our professions to the promising youth of the country. In advertising for prospective student nurses, we see too much emphasis placed on the salary, security, and prestige elements and too little on looking after the sick.

Other approaches used in dealing with personnel shortages are likely to tread on professional toes left sticking too far out in aisles traveled by the public. We must find additional ways to use auxiliary aides and volunteers and learn to weld them more securely into our professional team. Extensively trained professionals must work more exclusively in the jobs for which they were trained. We need to be certain that our professional boundary lines are not so fixed that it becomes impossible to deal with life situations. For example, in some areas of rural Canada the manifold problems arising among a very scattered rural population are probably going to require the development of a sort of combined public health nurse and social worker. Neither nursing training nor social work training has gone on sufficiently long compared to the history of man on this planet to give a legitimate feeling that the final answer is at hand. Freedom must be left for future experimentation.

Close physical proximity of various professional workers to each other and to the neighborhood in which they work is the basis for the health center concept. A health center makes it possible for all members of the family to find the needed health facilities and services more or less under a single roof. At any rate, people in the center can serve as guides to whatever services are needed in addition to those furnished. The definitive health center is probably not yet in existence, but its elements are to be found in various places.

The Peckham Pioneer Health Center in London is making

very important contributions, especially as a biological research center, for which it was founded, and has helped point the way toward broader possibilities. I am sure, however, that Dr. Innes Pearse and Dr. G. Scott Williamson do not feel they have yet found the absolute final answer. Interesting experiments will be going on in various parts of England in connection with the new National Health Service. South Africa is advancing some important concepts, and in many places in this country we can see health centers operating on varying plans.

In the English city of Manchester, "town planners have developed quite definite ideas on the relationship of the health center and the community center to a living neighborhood." They plan for homogenous neighborhoods of 10,000 people, and "within the neighborhood centre are sited the main shopping groups, the health sub-centre, community centre, branch library, two public houses and a church. The community centre and modern school are placed close together so that some of their accommodation may be interchangeable." [7] Closer coördination of health center and community center planning is highly desirable, just as the health council is probably more effective when functioning as part of a broad community council than when it acts alone.

Students of community anatomy and physiology will want to see our health professions organized into some sort of a recognizable structure. The Community Service Society's pattern has certain definite advantages and shows how numerous health and welfare activities may be united under a single administrative head. As a volunteer agency, its record of flexibility and clearheaded experimentation is remarkable. There have been broad vision and full acceptance of the obligation to train others. However, it is doubtful if this pattern of a broad voluntary agency can be applied on a community-wide basis throughout the nation. A very large proportion of the national need must be met by governmental agencies and by the individual initiative of private physicians. We must, therefore, recognize an element of artificiality in the Community Service Society method of inte-

[7] R. Nicholas, *City of Manchester Plan* (London: Jarrold & Sons, 1945), p. 139.

grating services, though this detracts very little from its value as an important laboratory for social experimentation. Any laboratory introduces, more or less, elements of artificiality.

At the Federal level we are likely to see the enactment soon of legislation establishing a cabinet department of health, education, and security. Medical and public health organizations have long sought a separate Federal department of health, but achievement of this now seems unlikely. There are excellent reasons for coördination of the three fields in a single department of the Federal Government. At this level where broad planning, gathering of data, controlled experimentation, and consultation between various technical groups would be the main functions rather than an operating program providing actual services to the people, there is more reason to favor this unification than to oppose it.

In the state and local governments, there are only isolated examples of a combined health and welfare department, and I know of none in which education is also a component part. Where the agency personnel actually serve the people, there is more present reason for separate administrative organization than for combinations so large that they become unwieldy. At the operating level we must gather together the services most closely related to health and group them together in a single administration, staffing the agency with personnel whose training is especially directed along health lines. Education has health interests, it is true, and they need opportunity for development and improvement, but the major concern is general education, and the necessary staff members have a specialized training and employ techniques differing from those of most health workers. Welfare activities also have very close relationships with health, including recreation and the various forms of social security, but welfare workers too have different skills and techniques. In our present stage of development, there are advantages in having separate agencies for health, education, and welfare at the operating level. But with this separation, we must keep clear lines of communication open in both directions.

Reasons for preserving the voluntary agencies working in

health, welfare, and recreation are well known and do not require discussion at this time. It is sufficient to say that they are essential parts of the picture so long as they integrate their work into the broad needs of the community. Most important contributions are also made by private practitioners and groups of practitioners working in the various fields. The element of free competition has certain advantages of which we must not lose sight. However, unless the independent operator is fully aware of community facilities and knows how to use them, he is depriving his clients or patients of the best sort of care available. The day of the little black bag, whether it be carried by physician or public health nurse, has passed, if we expect all the elements of a comprehensive family health program to be contained within such narrow confines.

Though it might simplify planning, I think we must agree that it is administratively unwise to place all our community activities concerned with health in a single agency. It is preferable to make adequate provision for joint planning, leaving the execution to the various agencies best qualified to work in the fields involved. The community council with its special committees on health, child care, family welfare, group work, etc., is the best mechanism for joint planning yet developed. Problems in the health field are dealt with by the health committee or council, which must have a considerable degree of autonomy if it is to be really effective. Representation of all important voluntary and official health interests must be complete, and consumers should also have an adequate voice. Financial support for the council is provided best from voluntary funds, such as the community chest. The value of such councils lies in their power of persuasion and community pressure rather than coercion. For any degree of success, active participation of governmental agencies is essential. This occurs only if representatives of these agencies are free to express themselves. They must not be made to feel that the council is trying to determine the final policies of the governmental agencies. It is important to recall that representatives of official agencies are likely to be in the minority around the council table since voluntary agencies are usually more numerous in the community even though the services rendered may be slight and the budget small compared to the governmental activities and expenditures. If the council is really representative of community leadership, it will have sufficient influence to make its weight felt even without the power to enforce its decisions.

I am sure you realize that I have no new system of team play to propose, no razzle-dazzle to replace emphasis on fundamentals. Each of us must understand, not only his own assignments, but what his teammates are doing as well. Everything possible must be done to make our services available to the family with a minimum of lost motion and friction. Planning and experimentation must be continuing.

While the team is important, each one of us must have our own ever expanding vision of the job we can do. "Before we can get the ways and means of bringing about a new world, we must first get people who believe that a new world is possible. New techniques will not succeed; a new soul, a new faith, are what we must have." [8] These are the words of the chaplain of Smith College. We may expend vast sums of money in providing hospitals, health centers, and clinics and in paying all sorts of workers; we may plan and plan for productive professional interplay; and we may study the needs and desires of families we are to serve. Some good will come from all this; but unless the members of our team are real people themselves with well-adjusted lives motivated by high purpose, any success we may have will be limited indeed.

[8] William G. Cole, "The World Needs to Find Its Soul," *Smith Alumnae Quarterly*, XXXIX (February, 1948), 65–67.

A Public Health Program as a Major Community Service

C.-E. A. WINSLOW, DR.P.H.

PUBLIC HEALTH AND PUBLIC WELFARE represent the two most powerful, practical forces for good in the evolution of modern society. They are intimately related; and their mutual interactions have been strikingly illustrated in the history of the Community Service Society of New York and in that of the two organizations which merged to form that society, the Association for Improving the Condition of the Poor and the Charity Organization Society.

The hundredth anniversary of the Community Service Society is dated from the formal incorporation of the Association for Improving the Condition of the Poor on December 14, 1848; but the inception of the agency actually goes even further back, to the year 1843 when plans were made for this pioneer organization and Robert Hartley was appointed its agent. The program was based on the concept that, while almsgiving must precede health care, those who would meet the "progressive exigencies" of the poor as well as "relieve their existing necessity" must devise a system by which the means for restoring health can move hand in hand with "relief of the poverty which most often results from illness."

In 1845 the Association called attention to the "wretched sanitary conditions of the tenement houses"; and in 1846, a year before the organization of the American Medical Association, the Association districted the city and organized a "system for the supply of the indigent sick with gratuitous medical aid." Thus, before the Association for Improving the Condition of the

Poor was actually incorporated, it had begun an attack on the two problems of public health that are most urgent in 1948—housing and medical care.

The Community Service Society has assembled an admirable summary of the historical development of the work of the A.I.C.P., the C.O.S., and the C.S.S.; but there is one intriguing question to which I have not found an answer—the origin of the name of the original parent organization. John Simon, in his first annual report as Health Officer of the City of London in 1847, wrote this pregnant sentence: "I feel the deepest conviction that no sanitary system can be adequate to the requirements of the time, or can cure those radical ills which infest the underframework of society unless the importance be distinctly recognized, and the duty manfully undertaken, of improving the social condition of the poor." Can this identity of phraseology be accidental? Or did Hartley chance to read Simon's report? Or was the A.I.C.P. operating under that name prior to 1848, and did Simon hear something of its work and adopt New York terminology in his London report? In any case, the story of these early years is one of the most inspiring examples of precocious vision in the history of public health.

In 1851 the A.I.C.P. opened the De Milt Dispensary, at Second Avenue and East 23d Street, where medical services were made available for poor persons living in that district; and established at Mott and Grand Streets the first public bath in the United States, "combining every convenience for bathing, washing, and ironing, at charges so low as to bring its advantages within the reach of all."

In the next year, 1852, another dispensary was opened on West 36th Street (it was called the "Northwestern Dispensary," a term which would scarcely be suitable today); and a committee appointed to inquire into the "sanitary conditions of the dwellings occupied by the laboring classes" reported that providing "the laboring classes with better tenements, improved ventilation and healthy and cleanly arrangements with respect to yards, sinks and sewerage will result in less sickness and premature mortality among them as well as fewer victims of disease among the more fortunate residents of the city." In 1855 the Working Men's Home Association, organized by the A.I.C.P., erected a model tenement for eighty-seven Negro families at Mott and Elizabeth Streets.

At this time, too, the Association took an active part in the movement for reform in the local public health service. Mr. Hartley testified at Albany in favor of the bill for a sanitary commission in New York City (1858)—legislation which has formed the cornerstone for public health administrative practice in the United States; and in 1862 the A.I.C.P. fostered the first New York State legislation for the improvement of milk supplies.

The first public health nursing service in the home on this continent was provided by the Women's Branch of the New York City Mission in 1877; and in 1878 the A.I.C.P. utilized City Mission nurses and a nurse employed by the Ethical Culture Society for home care in its families and for service in connection with the De Milt Dispensary.

In 1882 the Charity Organization Society was incorporated and took its place alongside the A.I.C.P. as a fellow worker in a common cause. Both organizations established offices in the new United Charities Building at Fourth Avenue and East 22d Street. In 1893, the A.I.C.P. opened the Sea Side Home for Crippled and Ailing Children on Coney Island; and developed its home services in teaching home nursing, child care, and homemaking. Both organizations actively supported the establishment of a tuberculosis sanatorium in the Adirondacks. The C.O.S. created an active committee for tenement house reform and advocated (1898) a system by "which persons of moderate incomes may pay regular dues as in a friendly society" and when in need obtain "medical attendance free or for a nominal sum."

In the first decade of the present century the C.O.S. employed district nurses to "devote their entire time to the care of sick patients who are under treatment at home and to teaching the patients themselves and other members of their families how to care for those who are to remain at home." The A.I.C.P. initiated a special advisory service for pregnant women and employed a visiting housekeeper to assist in homes handicapped by sickness.

The Milbank Memorial Bath was opened in 1904. In 1905 the A.I.C.P. embarked on an intensive campaign for public education in hygiene through "printed propaganda." In 1906 it organized the New York Milk Committee. In 1907 it developed a "well-organized prenatal nursing service."

The decade between 1910 and 1919 was notable for the continuing evolution of the role of the public health nurse as a teacher of health in the home, in which the Department of Educational Nursing of the A.I.C.P.—and the C.S.S.—has played a leading role.

In 1917 a C.O.S. committee made a study of illness in 103 families and pointed out that 55 percent of the illness was of a chronic or degenerative type "in which the individual needs re-education and adaptation to lead an efficient life and where the social and economic situation must be understood in order to improve conditions." Meanwhile, tuberculosis control received earnest attention; and in 1919 the C.O.S. Committee for the Prevention of Tuberculosis became the New York Tuberculosis and Health Association. In the same year dental hygiene became an active part of the program.

It is impossible to review the developments of more recent years in detail. Nutrition, home economics, and mental hygiene play increasingly important parts in the picture. Throughout the years between 1848 (or really 1843) and 1939, the A.I.C.P. and the C.O.S. have demonstrated a vision and a pioneering courage which are truly astounding. There is scarcely an important phase of modern public health in which these organizations have not been among the first in the field; and initiative has been balanced by wisdom which has insured soundness and has continuously evolved techniques which have been accepted as models throughout the United States and in foreign lands.

It was in 1939 that these two organizations, the A.I.C.P. and the C.O.S., which had rendered such notably distinguished service joined forces and merged into the Community Service Society of New York to pool their experiences in helping families to maintain or regain the power of self-help even though "beset by such difficulties as sickness, unemployment, marital conflict and mental breakdown."

Words are important things when they embody ideas; and the historical evolution of public welfare is thrown into sharp relief by the titles of the three organizations we have considered. In 1848, the emphasis on "improving the condition of the poor" reflected an urgent realization of the stark need of the underprivileged. How that need was to be met, the A.I.C.P. was to determine empirically through its pioneering years. A third of a century later, when the C.O.S. was incorporated, it was clear that "organization," organization of community resources and services, was the order of the day. In 1939, the merger was effected under the banners of the words "community" and "service."

"The poor" and the concept of "charity" were not forgotten. Yet today we recognize that the need for social services is not limited to the submerged tenth. It is a vital aid to healthful and efficient and satisfying living at all levels on the economic scale. It is an essential community service.

Furthermore, the stress on the word "service" is of profound significance. In 1913, when a generous gift from Mrs. Elizabeth Milbank Anderson made possible great expansion of the health program of the A.I.C.P., that association was reorganized to include two separate departments—the Department of Social Welfare to promote and to conduct research, study and demonstration programs adequate "to strike at the fundamental causes of poverty"; and the Department of Family Welfare "to coördinate its work of family rehabilitation, its personal service, its fresh air work, its educational nursing, its instruction of expectant mothers and its teaching of home economy."

This was an early recognition of the fact that in the over-all fields of public health and public welfare there are two more or less distinct essentials. The first of these is the provision of the broad community facilities which "strike at the fundamental causes of poverty" and disease. The functioning of a well-organized health department, of a safe water supply and systems of waste disposal, the provision of hospital and clinic facilities, a sound public housing program, an adequate system of social security—all these are necessary backgrounds for our work. They must, in the main, be provided by the agencies of government or, in the case of hospitals and clinics, by special voluntary agencies. The A.I.C.P. and the C.O.S. and the C.S.S. have rendered yeoman service in campaigning for such services throughout the years. They must continue to do so in the future. In particular, continuing research and evaluation of such background facilities should be a primary responsibility of such an organization as the C.S.S. Governmental functions are apt to become standardized and static without the constant pioneering efforts of voluntary groups of citizens.

Effective coördination of public agencies and expansion into new emerging fields of public health and welfare have come in rich measure from the leadership of the A.I.C.P. and C.O.S. The C.S.S. is fully alive to the need for continued activities along this line, as evidenced by its Institute of Welfare Research and its Bureau of Public Affairs and its Committee on Housing. It is probable that such research and planning and stimulating functions are among the most valuable and the most lasting contributions of the voluntary health and welfare agencies.

Beyond the area of broad and fundamental community facilities, however, there lies a domain of direct counseling service to the individual family which has been another major contribution of the nonofficial agency. There is a considerable measure of overlapping here. The health department has its public health nurses, the hospital its medical social workers, the department of public assistance, its investigators. The primary initiative, particularly in the Eastern United States, has come from the voluntary agency. The C.S.S. operated in 1947 eleven district offices for family service, with 140 family caseworkers, fourteen homemakers, two home economists, two employment counselors, one vocational counselor, and eleven special caseworkers for unattached boys and men. In the Department of Educational Nursing, it maintained eight neighborhood offices with a staff of sixty-five public health nurses. All this was in addition to ten nutritionists and to the twenty-six nurses and hygienists and part-

Public Health Program and the Community

time doctors and dentists serving the clinics of the Society and the seven summer camps, three homes for the aged, and one "sheltered workshop" provided by the organization. If you can imagine what such expert counseling means to the individual family, not only to the "poor," but on all economic levels, you will realize how supremely important is such "service" for the "community" as a whole.

The annual report of the C.S.S. for 1945–46 was entitled "The Family a Force for Peace"; and this phrase admirably emphasizes the basic objective of the Society. We need, and in a more and more complex and crowded society we shall increasingly need, broad community facilities of various sorts for the foundations of our communal living. Yet if the good life is to be attained, these public and semipublic services must not be forced upon us. They must be understood and accepted by the people themselves. In such an understanding and acceptance, the family must be a basic factor. There are forces at work in modern society which have profoundly influenced the power of family tradition as it has been exercised in past generations; and some mitigation of a too overpowering familial authority is probably desirable. Brock Chisholm, the distinguished Canadian psychiatrist who now heads the secretariat of the World Health Organization, has pointed out that a major part of emotional maladjustment in the past has come from a sense of guilt due to conflict between individual possibilities and too rigid and arbitrary social and moral codes. He does not allude to the even greater menaces to emotional health which arise when a reasonable diversity of more or less similar family codes is replaced by a single uniform strait jacket of thought and feeling imposed by the state as a whole. The extraordinary confessions made in political trials under the Soviet regime are explicable only on the basis of a sense of guilt experienced under such a totalitarian regime.

There must, however, be channels of communication by means of which the lessons learned through earlier generations may be passed on to the citizens of the future; and the family—shorn of some of the arbitrary traditionalism of the past—is by far the most promising instrument for this purpose. In the family alone can such a message be effectively delivered, because by the time a child is exposed to the influence of the school and the Church, most of its emotional mind-sets have already been established. Here, the neurotic tendencies which cause wars and revolutions have, in the past, been nurtured. In the family, as Chisholm says,

> We were taught to be absolutely loyal and obedient to the local concept of virtue whatever that happened to be. We were taught that Moslems or Hindus or Jews, or Democrats or Republicans (with us in Canada, Grits or Tories) or capitalists or trade unionists, or socialists or communists, or Roman Catholics or Methodists or any of all other human groups are wrong or even wicked. It almost always happened that among all the people in the world only our own parents and perhaps a few people they selected, were right about everything. We could refuse to accept their rightness only at the price of a load of guilt and fear, and peril to our immortal souls. This training has been practically universal in the human race. Variations in content have had almost no importance. The fruit is poisonous no matter how it is prepared or disguised.[1]

What we must look forward to in the future is the replacement of arbitrary tribal codes by true education, the kind of education which aims at the molding of a free and responsible personality. Maturity, not crystallization of past mores, must be our objective; and what this implies has been well stated by Strecker and Appel. They tell us that

> Maturity is a quality of personality that is made up of a number of elements. It is stick-to-it-iveness, the ability to stick to a job, to work on it, and to struggle through until it is finished, or until one has given all one has in the endeavor. It is the quality or capacity of giving more than is asked or required in a given situation. It is this characteristic that enables others to count on one; thus it is reliability. Persistence is an aspect of maturity: persistence to carry out a goal in the face of difficulties. Endurance of difficulties, unpleasantness, discomfort, frustration, hardship. The ability to size things up, make one's own decision, is a characteristic of maturity. This implies a considerable amount of independence. A mature person is not dependent unless ill. Of course, maturity represents the capacity to coöperate: to work with others, to work in an organization and under authority. The mature person is flexible, can defer to time, persons,

[1] G. B. Chisholm, "The Reëstablishment of Peacetime Society," *Psychiatry*, IX, No. 1 (February, 1946), 8.

circumstances. He can show tolerance, he can be patient, and above all he has the qualities of adaptability and compromise. Basically, maturity represents a wholesome amalgamation of two things: (1) dissatisfaction with the *status quo,* which calls forth aggressive, constructive effort, and (2) social concern and devotion. It is morale in the individual.[2]

It is this new concept, of maturity rather than conformity, which must be cultivated in the homes of the future if our civilization is to survive. For the attainment of such an end, the home must be buttressed by such broad community facilities as have been discussed in earlier paragraphs; and particularly, it may be noted that our housing program lies at the very heart of the matter. Most modern social forces operate outside the home; but the provision of decent dwelling accommodations tends to balance the scale and make the life of a family a real and a vital and a continuing force for good.

In any case, the provision of common facilities must be supplemented and infused by an educational process which inspires and guides the individual family to play its part in the task of communal living. It is here that the stress of the C.S.S. on educational service in the home is of such supreme importance. The 1945–46 report states that "the family is a 'shock absorber of social change' in the daily experience of every C.S.S. staff member." It notes that in emerging from the strains of war, the family faced its own peculiarly acute problems:

War-wedded couples, many with children, found their first opportunity to take up life together and to practice the delicate art of family relationships; reunited families faced the inevitable adjustments involved in settling down again to the every day responsibilities of making a home. And it was these new and reunited families who were the most harassed by housing shortages, mounting prices and countless uncertainties.[3]

The report continues,

Timely therefore was the Society's emphasis on service to children, young people and young married couples, for on them rests the fu-

[2] Edward A. Strecker and Kenneth E. Appel, *Psychiatry in Modern Warfare* (New York: Macmillan, 1945), pp. 70–71.

[3] "The Family a Force for Peace," Annual Report of the Community Service Society of New York, 1945–1946 (New York: C.S.S., 1947), p. 7.

ture of the American home. The sound bodies, minds and hearts so urgently needed for the world we now live in must be nurtured in the family. The strong family can be a strong force for peace. In these days the Society's basic goal of strengthening the family—of sustaining and enhancing the values of family life—is fraught with heightened significance.[4]

Individualized service to families is no less a function of the Department of Educational Nursing under the direction of Alta E. Dines. This service is intensive and reaches only a small number of families (2,664 in the last fiscal year). Its objective is the type of health teaching fitted to the individual family needs and situations which every good public health nurse wants to do but which is difficult to accomplish in any covering service or in a numerically heavy service. Group work supplements family teaching and is developed around need and readiness; classes, conferences, demonstrations, workshops, even parties may fit the special needs of an age group, a particular social or ethnic group.

Well-qualified, experienced public health nurses are eligible for this staff, and they are chosen because of special interest and aptitudes. They are only partially prepared for this type of health teaching. They always need a considerable period of orientation to this agency and time to develop their educational skills for successful application to family and community situations. The health concept seems difficult to understand; for therapy is more stressed than education; diseases, their cure and prevention, are more prominent than health in the so-called "health programs" in which nurses have participated.

Several features of this health nursing service have been repeatedly singled out for comment by students from many universities and countries. For instance:

1. The family is the unit of service: every individual in the family is a matter of concern for needed curative services, for health examinations with interpretation and follow-up; the whole family is included when the health nurse teaches housekeeping for health, budgeting for health, recreation for health, food for health.

[4] *Ibid.*, pp. 7–8.

2. Health counseling is an important part of service to the family: helping the members of the family to learn what they do not already know about keeping well; helping the family know and select wisely for use the community medical and health facilities in relation to their quality and the family's economic status; helping the family to select and read available health literature.

3. The emphasis is on depth and comprehensiveness of service rather than quantity.

In the Community Service Society nursing department, the program is flexible, fitted to individual, to family, to groups, to community, on the basis of the urgency of the presenting need, of the ability of the staff to give the indicated service, and, of course, on the suitability of the Society's participation in such a service and the implications. Whenever feasible, the department shares in studies or research projects which aim at increasing knowledge about family health, how it can be attained and safeguarded.

Such a program as this—even if it serves at present only a few thousand families—is of profound significance for the philosophy of living in these troublous times. It is the seedbed of the future.

Social planning on a wide and comprehensive scale is essential for survival in the complex and changing world in which we live. We must firmly reject the two extreme philosophies which so largely dominate the political thinking of the present day. One of these philosophies is totalitarianism. It sees so clearly the dangers of drift that it turns to complete domination by the State as the only remedy. We must all be totalitarian in wartime. The objectives of winning a war are simple and defined, and the immediate peril is so great that the end justifies the means. But the objectives of peace are broader and more complex. They cannot be crystallized. They change from day to day. Only a free choice by mature men can solve them. Embodiment in the static, revealed religion of a Marxian code can only lead to the catastrophe which overcame the giant saurians of an earlier geologic age; and rigidity under the State will inevitably lead to those emotional conflicts which lie at the root of individual and mass neuroses.

Nor can the opposite philosophy of anarchistic individualism yield any more adequate solution of our common problem. This, too, is based on an arbitrary and inadequate abstraction, on the religious dogma of *laissez faire*, the touching faith that if everyone fights vigorously enough against everyone else, some mystic law will bring everything out all right in the end. This is a philosophy which worships the individual, as totalitarianism worships the State. Neither unrestrained individual selfishness nor blind submission to authority can solve the problems of the modern world.

The only answer can be found, in the State, as in the family, by the development of an attitude of maturity, which combines recognition of the sacredness of the individual with recognition of common obligations to society. It is this sort of attitude which the Community Service Society is developing; and the stimulation of mature thinking through educational leadership can be performed with peculiar success by a voluntary organization of this type which has no power of compulsion but must base its leadership solely on the convincing power of its ideals and its comprehension of the realities of life.

Can we solve the problems of the world by developing an adequate degree of maturity, a broad enough base of coöperation for the common good, by free men and women acting deliberately of their own free will in the general interest of mankind? Can we do it in time? Can our grasp of the science of human living be brought level with our astounding mastery over physical forces which are equally available for the enrichment or destruction of mankind? We do not know the answer to this question. But we know where the one avenue of salvation lies.

A visitor to a modern institution for the care of advanced cases of mental disease was startled to find a group of patients working on the grounds with a single guard sitting and smoking under a tree. The visitor said to the guard, "Aren't you afraid these crazy people might get together and do some harm?" "No," replied the guard, "I ain't afraid. Crazy people don't never get together."

The moral is obvious; and the challenge is acute.

Index of Articles and Contributing Authors

ACHIEVING FAMILY HEALTH THROUGH MODERN EDUCATION, Ernest Osborne, 252
Ackerman, Nathan W., M.D., Director, Council Child Development Center, New York, N.Y.; "The Adaptive Problems of the Adolescent Personality," 85
ADAPTIVE PROBLEMS OF THE ADOLESCENT PERSONALITY, THE, Nathan W. Ackerman, M.D., 85
ADOLESCENCE—ITS IMPLICATIONS FOR FAMILY AND COMMUNITY, Viola W. Bernard, M.D., 121
ADOLESCENCE IN OUR SOCIETY, Harold E. Jones, 70

Bernard, Viola W., M.D., Consultant on Adolescents to Family Service, Community Service Society of New York; Associate in Psychiatry, College of Physicians and Surgeons, Columbia University, New York, N.Y.; "Adolescence—Its Implications for Family and Community," 121
Burke, Bertha S., Assistant Professor of Maternal and Child Nutrition, Department of Maternal and Child Health, School of Public Health, Harvard University, Boston, Mass.; "The Next Generation—Its Nutrition and Health," 204
Burns, Eveline M., Professor of Social Work, New York School of Social Work, Columbia University, New York, N.Y.; "Economic Factors in Family Life," 12

Burritt, Bailey B., Executive Secretary, Health Maintenance Committee, Community Service Society of New York, New York, N.Y.; formerly Executive Director, National Health Council, New York, N.Y.; "Maintenance of Health: Exploring in New York," 183

CHILD HEALTH IN RELATION TO THE FAMILY, Martha Eliot, M.D., and Neota Larson, 159
CHILD REARING IN THE CLASS STRUCTURE OF AMERICAN SOCIETY, W. Allison Davis, 56
CONSTRUCTIVE MEDICINE AND POSITIVE HEALTH, Henry E. Meleney, M.D., 198

Davis, W. Allison, Associate Professor of Education, University of Chicago, Chicago, Ill.; "Child Rearing in the Class Structure of American Society," 56
Dollard, John, Research Associate in Human Relations, Institute of Human Relations, Yale University, New Haven, Conn.; "Do We Have a Science of Child Rearing?" 41
DO WE HAVE A SCIENCE OF CHILD REARING? John Dollard, 41
Dublin, Thomas D., M.D., Dr. P.H. Executive Director, National Health Council, New York, N.Y.; "Health and Family Life: Health Maintenance," 194

Index of Articles and Authors

ECONOMIC FACTORS IN FAMILY LIFE, Eveline M. Burns, 12

Eliot, Martha, M.D., Associate Chief, United States Children's Bureau, Federal Security Agency, Washington, D.C.; Special Technical Consultant, International Children's Emergency Fund of the United Nations; President, American Public Health Association, New York, N.Y.; "Child Health in Relation to the Family," 159

FOOD FOR THE FAMILY OF NATIONS, F. Verzar, 229

French, Thomas M., M.D., Associate Director, Institute for Psychoanalysis, Chicago, Ill.; "Personal Interaction and Growth in Family Life," 29

HEALTH AND FAMILY LIFE: HEALTH MAINTENANCE, Thomas D. Dublin, M.D., Dr. P.H., 194

Hubbard, Ruth W., General Director, Visiting Nurse Society of Philadelphia, Philadelphia, Pa.; President, National Organization for Public Health Nursing, New York, N.Y.; "Nursing for Health in Tomorrow's Family," 242

Jones, Harold E., Director, Institute of Child Welfare, University of California, Berkeley, Calif.; "Adolescence in Our Society," 70

King, Charles Glen, Scientific Director, Nutrition Foundation, New York, N.Y.; Professor of Chemistry, Columbia University, New York, N.Y.; "Nutrition in the Home and in the Community, 221

Kluckhohn, Clyde, Director, Russian Research Center, Harvard University, Cambridge, Mass.; "Variations in the Human Family," 3

Kris, Ernst, Visiting Professor of Psychology, New School for Social Research and College of the City of New York, New York, N.Y.; "Roots of Hostility and Prejudice," 141

Larson, Neota, Assistant to the Associate Chief, United States Children's Bureau, Federal Security Agency, Washington, D.C.; "Child Health in Relation to the Family," 159

Leavell, Hugh R., M.D., Dr. P.H., Professor of Public Health Practice, School of Public Health, Harvard University, Boston, Mass.; "Professional Interplay for Family Health," 263

MAINTENANCE OF HEALTH: EXPLORING IN NEW YORK, Bailey B. Burritt, 183

Meleney, Henry E., M.D., Herman M. Biggs Professor of Preventive Medicine, College of Medicine, New York University, New York, N.Y.; "Constructive Medicine and Positive Health," 198

NEXT GENERATION—ITS NUTRITION AND HEALTH, THE, Bertha S. Burke, 204

NURSING FOR HEALTH IN TOMORROW'S FAMILY, Ruth W. Hubbard, 242

NUTRITION IN THE HOME AND IN THE COMMUNITY, Charles Glen King, 221

Osborne, Ernest, Professor of Education, Teachers College, Columbia University, New York, N.Y.; "Achieving Family Health through Modern Education," 252

Pearse, Innes H., M.D., Medical Director, Pioneer Health Center (Peckham Experiment), London, England; "Pioneering in London: the Peckham Experiment," 170

PERSONAL INTERACTION AND GROWTH IN FAMILY LIFE, Thomas M. French, M.D., 29

PIONEERING IN LONDON: THE PECKHAM EXPERIMENT, Innes H. Pearse, M.D., 170

PROFESSIONAL INTERPLAY FOR FAMILY HEALTH, Hugh R. Leavell, M.D., Dr. P.H., 263

PUBLIC HEALTH PROGRAM AS A MAJOR COMMUNITY SERVICE, A, C.-E. A. Winslow, Dr. P.H., 273

ROOTS OF HOSTILITY AND PREJUDICE, Ernst Kris, 141

Index of Articles and Authors

VARIATIONS IN THE HUMAN FAMILY, Clyde Kluckhohn, 3

Verzar, F., Acting Director, Nutrition Division, Food and Agriculture Organization of the United Nations; "Food for the Family of Nations," 229

Winslow, C.-E. A., Dr. P. H., Professor Emeritus of Public Health, Yale University, New Haven, Conn.; Editor, *American Journal of Public Health;* "A Public Health Program as a Major Community Service," 273

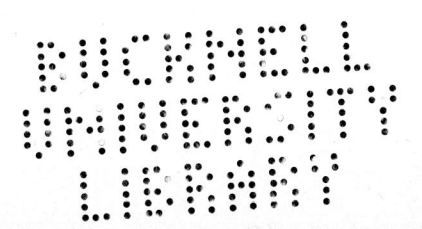